TWICE

HOW I BECAME A CANCER-SLAYING
SUPER MAN BEFORE I TURNED 21

by Benjamin Rubenstein

Illustrated by
Anthony Geist

Tree,

To Health!

Benin. Rubens

Woodley Books

Text © Copyright Benjamin Rubenstein 2010.
Interior illustrations and design © Copyright 2010 by Woodley Books, LLC
All rights reserved. No portion of this book may be reproduced or utilized
in any form or by any electronic, mechanical, or other means
without the prior written permission of the publishers.
Printed in the United States of America.
Published by Woodley Books, LLC.
Cover design: Anthony Geist/Ghosthousestudios.com
Interior design: Sherry Charles/Where Books Begin
Cataloguing-in-Publication Data.
Rubenstein, Benjamin.
Twice: How I Became A Cancer-Slaying Super Man
Before I Turned 21 by Benjamin Rubenstein.
ISBN 1. Rubenstein, Benjamin-Health.
2. Cancer-Patients-United States-Biography.
3. Cancer-Humor.
RC 265.6 S29A3 2010
362,196
10 9 8 7 6 5 4 3 2 1 1 0 1 1 1 2 1 3 1 4
ISBN: 978-0-9786472-9-2

For permissions and further information contact:
Woodley Books
204 E. Broad St.
Bethlehem, PA 18018
www.woodleybooks.com
484-274-6841
Customer.service@woodleybooks.com

All of the events and people described in this book are real.
To protect the privacy of the people who saved my life, I have
changed names and circumstances at their requests. However, some people
wanted to be acknowledged as part of my story and so I have retained
their real names and circumstances here. Sort it out for yourself,
but be assured this story is absolutely true.

In memory of
Matthew David Cole and
Charles Franklin Fletcher III

TABLE OF

CONTENTS

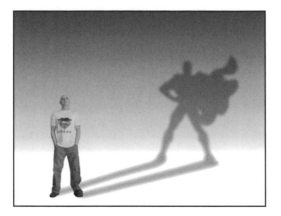

CANCER: MY OWN PERSONAL PHONE BOOTH

I keep a photo in my wallet of myself before I got cancer. The photo had been taken right before I began treatment, a symbol of who I used to be, who I could have continued being if it hadn't been for that uncontrolled group of cells. That boy is now like a favorite dead relative.

One day a friend asked to look at it. "This was when you were sixteen?" she asked, grinning at my youthful appearance. "Do you look at it often?"

"No," I replied, snatching the picture from her. But before I stuffed it back in my wallet, I stared at the teenage boy looking back at me. He was a talented tennis player, a good student, a Hebrew teacher at the synagogue, a loving son and an adoring brother. This sixteen-year-old Benjamin was living happily in Manassas, Virginia in a town full of friends and family and even though he was too short to be a heartbreaker, girls loved his hair.

This teenage Benjamin was completely unprepared for cancer. All he knew was the treatment for cancer made people lose their hair. He didn't know anything about how cancer changed people's outlooks. As he learned about cancer, he also began learning about himself. That kid in the photo in my wallet saved my life. I love that kid.

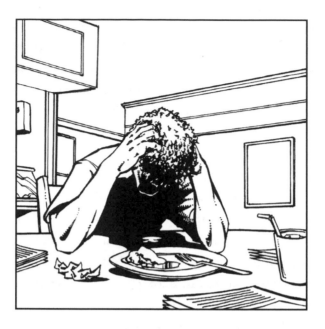

Chapter 1
FOREVER SIXTEEN

I liked being sixteen. If time was to stop and I could be stuck at one age for the rest of my life, even now I would want to stay sixteen forever. The only two drawbacks were not being legally able to get into an R-rated movie, and the hip thing.

On my sixteenth birthday, a cold, dark night in December—when I hopped in my car, I was alone, for the first time. I filled the twelve-disc CD changer my parents had bought me for my birthday with a few of my all-time favorites. I wanted to cruise to nowhere in particular. The freedom that came with sixteen was a powerful thing. I no longer had to wait for my mom to take me to Best Buy to buy that new CD. I was no longer just a kid. I no longer needed a ride to hang out with friends.

I didn't have a girlfriend, though I was keeping an eye on Lily

McGrath. I did have quite a few friends, like Andy Hardin, with whom I played a lot of *Super Tennis* on Super Nintendo. When the game *Perfect Dark* came out Andy and I played it eleven consecutive hours, with a short dinner break. My oldest friend, from birth, was Drew Thornton but Andy was the one I watched *Half-Baked* with, and tried to locate shots of Mandy Moore's ass. I had pals at school, too, including Bently, Nick Linebaugh and Worm. I was sixteen without a care in the world, except how to seduce Lily without having to talk to her.

Early on, I showed signs of gifted intelligence, so my parents had high expectations of me academically. By sixteen, there was a little rift between me and my mom because I wasn't meeting those expectations. I was taking AP classes in history and English but grades were not my top priority as they had been with her. My mom had always been at the head of her class.

On the other hand, my dad was pretty laid-back, at least when he was at home with my big brother Jonathan and me. Jonathan and I would often call my dad by one of his many nicknames: Carrot, Bull's Eye, Pudding, Pooper Scooper, or any variation such as The Bull, Chocolate Pudding, or Pooper. He would even fart in public. "Wait a second... you'll be sitting at your desk with someone else in the office and just fart?" I asked him.

"Yeah, why not? What do I care?"

"I don't know, it's just weird. What does the other person do?"

"Usually just leaves."

"What if it's mid-conversation? Does he say anything?"

"No. If it's important, he'll come back. That's all."

I didn't study much but I played a lot of tennis. My friend Friedman was my doubles partner. I would have to constantly calm him down, tell him to chill. A year after I got cancer, Friedman would be #2 on the varsity team, and I tell him that should've been me because I'm better than him though I will never play again.

In singles competition, Friedman had the most powerful serve of any opponent I had faced. The year I was sixteen, we were battling for a spot on the varsity tennis team. Friedman was a technical player and I was a pusher, meaning I chased down every shot and hit the ball in play without worrying about placement. So long as I could run to the ball, I always had a chance to win. I was trying to win the day I felt a pain in my groin.

The pain was sharp, deep inside my hip, so deep that my mind couldn't pinpoint where it came from. The pain was simultaneous with my left Adidas's contact with the court. The only thing that I had experienced like it was my arousal to the first naked woman I saw in *Under Siege*. My eyes saw her, my prick rose. The difference was that time my boner had gone away. This pain did not.

I pushed through the pain because the season just begun. This couldn't be happening on the first day of practice. Over the coming months, other players jokingly called me a pussy. I started to wonder if I was a pussy. I also wondered if my tennis skills were diminishing, or if the new $80 racket I bought was worse than my old $20 piece of shit.

When I drove home later that evening my hip throbbed. It got worse.

A week later I found that running was becoming next to impossible. By the summer, I noticed a permanent bruise in my lower back. As summer dragged on, a tiny bulge emerged next to it. Within weeks, I was feeling pain going up steps. At my cousin's Bat Mitzvah even walking across the room hurt. Then I could barely walk at all.

I called Jonathan at Virginia Tech and he encouraged me to tell my parents about my pain. I knew it would be easy to see a doctor, but I wanted to wait until after our trip to Israel.

This trip was a big deal for us, a family vacation. My mom was a social worker, and my dad was a Federal employee. Our summer vacations usually consisted of a couple of amusement parks, some boring museums and the beach. They weren't my mom's ideal vacation, which

is why she'd been looking forward to this Israel trip for years. We were going to do it. I couldn't ruin it.

Our tour group met in Jerusalem and included an Olympic soccer goalie. We walked down Ben Yehuda Street with all the bars and shops. I bought a white t-shirt with the Superman shield wearing a black top hat and Hasidic earlocks that read "Super-Jew." Even though it got rave reviews from my friends, I was too embarrassed to wear it in public. The shirt stayed in my drawer, collecting powers.

When we climbed Mount Masada, on the Dead Sea, most of the group took the lift up to the top of the mountain. I decided to go with those who walked it in the 115-degree heat. "Are you sure you want to do this?" Jonathan said. "It'll be hard, even for me."

"No way am I sitting this one out."

After the forty-five minute climb, though, I felt a pain that even Cal Ripken, Jr., would respect me for pushing aside. On our final night in Israel, we played soccer. I, rather than the Olympian, was goalie. "When we get home I'll see the doctor and get it fixed. It's probably just a stress fracture," I promised Jonathan.

I went to the doctor the week after we got back. He asked a lot of questions but once I explained where the pain began—on the tennis court—he ordered an MRI, a magnetic body scan that can detect tumors. The radiologist studied the internal structures of my torso, contrasting between my different tissues. The MRI was for my back, but the radiologist saw a massive abnormality in the corner.

He ordered a second MRI to focus on that corner, without telling me that he saw a tumor there. Before he could prescribe a bone scan, the radiologist had to verify that I had an adolescent bone tumor which the second MRI showed. It took three weeks to schedule me for that second MRI. While we waited, the malignant cancer destroyed more of my bone. The bone scan was expedited as soon as they saw the results of the second MRI.

The next day I was in the lab for the bone scan. What a job it must have been for the bone scan technician. She saw my cancerous future in perfect clarity on her computer screen—a bright white spot over my left hip. But she didn't say a word, just smiled sweetly at me, and sent the results to the orthopedic surgeon.

The day of my appointment with the surgeon, Andy wanted to hang out after school, so I told him I had to see the surgeon. "What do you think he'll say?" Andy asked.

"He'll probably say my pain is from growing child-bearing hips."

My mom picked me up and took me to the appointment. The surgeon had me stand up and face away from him, butt naked underneath my gown, and he pushed my pelvic bone for over a minute. "Just say it's a stress fracture. Quit fucking with me," I thought, but didn't say it aloud more for my mom than for myself.

"Something is definitely growing there," he said. While I dressed, he talked to Mom. When we left I asked her, "What is it?"

"I'll tell you at home."

"What does 'growing' mean?"

"Please, Benjamin. I have to concentrate on this traffic. We'll talk about it when we get home."

The ride home was the longest twenty minutes of my life. The word "cancer" scrolled through my brain over and over, but it scrolled too fast to register. She dropped me off in front and went to park the car. I waited at the kitchen table for her, my leg twitching nervously. She gave it to me straight: "Benjamin, you have a tumor."

Boom! Those four words split my life into two distinctly different phases. Phase I was Pre-Cancer Ben: my first sixteen years, eight months, fourteen days and sixteen hours of life. Phase II began with, "You have a tumor," and will end the day I die. After a long pause she said, "Are you all right?"

"Yeah, I'm fine," I said. "Tumors are for Sick Kids. I'll never be fine

again," I thought to myself.

"No, you're not. I can see you're not fine."

"I'm going downstairs."

I was on the brink of tears. I called Drew. "Dude," I said in a choked voice, "I have something to tell you."

"What is it?"

"I have a tumor."

"Oh my God, I think I just shit myself."

Drew came over and we silently play *NFL Blitz 2000* on Nintendo 64. When my dad came home from work, he entered my room, walked in front of our game, kissed me on the forehead and left. I kept my eyes square with the TV, feeling the tension of three people who would rather be in Mogadishu. In case it was a false alarm I told Drew to keep it quiet. "I don't want to blow it out of proportion if it's nothing." A few days later I no longer cared how others found out. "Make somebody cry for me," I told Drew.

I don't know why I went to school the next day. I had been rocked by a life-altering uppercut and was now walking around the halls listening to people complaining about their girlfriends and asking how their jeans look.

After school I went into the computer room and cried for the first time in years. I tried to decide whether I should cry hard or just drip a few tears. My final decision was to go all-out: strange noises, head jerking, snot flow. As a teenager, I had been very focused on my groin ever since I had discovered how to extract my little swimmers while sunbathing on my patio. There was activity going on down there that interested me more than anything. I loved looking at girls, I liked to masturbate. So when I heard that I had a cancer growing near there, I was really deeply and totally alarmed. It wasn't like it was my liver or my lungs that I had never really had a relationship with. It was like dying myself plus having my best friend dying along with me. Would any girl be willing to blow

me now with a tumor there?

The tumor was located in my iliac crest and right next to the family jewels. The cancer, the disease, was alive, flourishing, invading my pelvic area, growing unabated right there. The blue, round-cell tumor hoarded my nourishment, crept through my hard bone, pushed against nerves and strong muscle fibers. It had been growing many months before I knew it was there, because there my pelvis provided so much room for growth. It wasn't just about my nuts; so many vital organs there depended on my white blood cells to seek and destroy the malignant cells, and would fail and die if smothered by the cancer.

My white cells did not attack, not because they were abnormal, but because they didn't perceive the cancer as a threat. The cells were me, not some alien organism, or foreign body, just an out-of-control replicating mass. The cells, known collectively as my tumor, were eight inches long. The cancer was me.

After a couple minutes, I felt awkward, so I stopped and vowed never to cry again. I had not cried the day before when Mom said I had a tumor, so why cry today? Why cry ever again?

The word was out. On Sunday morning when I went to Temple to teach Hebrew, the mother of a kid I had just finished tutoring for his Bar Mitzvah said, "Tell me what you know." I guessed my mom had told a few people.

"I don't know much. They don't know what it is yet, or if it's anything."

"What can I do for you?"

"Nothing, I'm fine. Thanks."

Like I said, when I turned sixteen, I was no longer a kid. I didn't need help or anyone to do anything for me. Within the first couple months of treatment I realized I was invincible. I saw myself as a real-life Super Man. Unable to be penetrated. Unable to be destroyed. It was a good thing that I reached this conclusion. I needed it to endure the long,

thin needle that entered my now softer-than-normal bone to retrieve a tumor sample to conclude if it was malignant or benign. In my head I already knew it was cancer. My pain got worse over the months, so it must be growing.

American track stars were on the TV when I stumbled into the waiting room for the biopsy. I didn't watch. The Summer Olympics in Sydney symbolized the peak of human performance, while I was being tortured with medical procedures to determine, effectively, how much longer I was supposed to live. I didn't care that Maurice Greene and Michael Johnson were about to win gold medals. The best summer of my life was ending catastrophically. I just wanted my enormous dose of Valium to make it all go away.

"I need to push through your bone, so you may hear the hammer. You might feel it, too. Let me know if it hurts," the biopsy technician said.

"I can hear the hammer pounding into my bone," I said laughing, elated. "Hey man, are you hungry?"

"Pretty hungry, yeah."

"I'm starving. When we're done, you and I are going to McDonald's, and my parents are treating." The Valium was making me manic. Of course we didn't go to McDonald's, he went to the next patient and I went home. Drew came over.

"Dude, you look so high right now," he said, seeing that the Valium hadn't quite worn off.

Without Valium, there wasn't much to laugh about. I became certain that the girls at school no longer saw me as the shy, quiet guy who drove his friends everywhere and made the occasional quip. I was convinced they saw me as a Sick Kid. I know this because that is how I would have viewed anyone else with cancer. I did everything in my power to show them otherwise. I've done everything I can since then, and I will do everything I can forever.

Many years later I saw a skiing documentary with my college

roommate, Tim. "How old do you think your skiing students are?" I asked Tim as we walked out of the theater.

"I think they're probably sixteen," my roommate said.

I couldn't believe it."They looked so young—like kids."

My roommate laughed. "Sixteen-year-olds are kids! Don't you remember?"

And that's when I recognized that we don't suddenly stop being kids when we turn sixteen. I didn't stop being a kid when I got cancer, even though I knew from the first diagnosis that Sweet Sixteen was over. I still say it was the best year of my life, perhaps never to be topped. There is something special about that age—maybe it's because my own life changed so dramatically then. Or, maybe it had something to do with my Super-Jew tee shirt.

By September, I was watching a never-ending parade of doctors at the National Institutes of Health (NIH) in Bethesda, Maryland. This behemoth hospital is only forty miles north of my parents' house but a world away from anything I had experienced before. The NIH Clinical Center was treating bone cancer on the pediatric floor. My cousin Elizabeth worked there as a researcher so when she heard I was sick, she had a doctor bypass the bureaucracy to get me in. My parents met with the doctors there without me a week before I was admitted and decided that would be a good place for me. While I cried alone, they were deciding where I would have the best chance of living past eighteen. We drove over to NIH during a school day for the first examination. We gathered around a large, round table where I sat next to my parents. "You have Ewing's sarcoma, a type of bone cancer," Dr. Springs, the first of the NIH doctors told me. Those files in my brain are corrupted and difficult to access. But I do remember how bad I felt.

Only about a hundred and fifty Americans are diagnosed with a Ewing's tumor each year, most between ten and twenty years old. That's

minuscule compared to the 200 thousand men diagnosed annually with prostate cancer. Ewing's sarcoma occurs more often in males than in females and the patients are predominantly white. Two-thirds survive more than five years. In my fantasy-addled mind, I thought it must be related to Patrick Ewing, the basketball player—I mean, how many Ewings can there be?

My parents made all the decisions about my treatment. My mom later told me she was nauseous and could barely talk but they maintained rational thought. In contrast, I couldn't stop obsessing about whether "sarcoma" began with an "s" or "c". Dr. Springs gave my parents forms to sign, authorizing different things, each basically stating, "Benjamin can die in this many different ways. We agree to this." The forms were explicit that I would vomit, receive blood transfusions, lose my curly hair (which I washed with girly shampoo twice a day) and become sterile. When he said there was a hundred percent chance I would be sterile, I said, "That sucks," the two words I could muster without crying. Even if I had not sworn never to cry again, I certainly didn't want to do it in front of my parents.

My family hid their pain well. After the surgeon announced that there was something growing in my pelvis, I sat outside his office, waiting for my mom to come out. I was frightened. Everyone was staring at me. I could hear the surgeon berate my mom, saying, "He has a lump. It doesn't do any good to hide your eyes. Everything points to cancer. You have to face it."

At home, my dad, when he felt the need to cry, went into another room. Even Jonathan, away at college, tried to sound tougher than he felt. "What are you telling me? Are you telling me that Benjamin is going to die?" he shouted over the phone when my mom broke the news to him.

My parents hid their anguish from me because the doctors at NIH had commanded them to, citing studies which claimed teenage patients coped better that way. My mom would forever wrestle with whether denial of their own pain was the right decision.

At the time, I wasn't thinking much of my family. I was barraged with information from so many doctors that I couldn't remember all their names. I retained the important stuff, mostly regarding length of time. Time before starting treatment. Time before ending treatment. Time between cycles. Time I'd miss school. What it really came down to was the time I would lose in my old life, and it would take time to get it back. What they couldn't tell me was how slow time would go. There was no way I could speed it up.

I wondered if I developed bone cancer by eating too much McDonald's and Burger King, but there was nothing I could have done. I never would have forgiven myself if I had caused a tumor. I still occasionally eat that crap, which hopefully won't produce a third nipple.

The floor treated children with HIV, cancer and skin diseases. I could navigate with my eyes shut. Exit the elevator, take a left through the sliding glass doors, and walk past the fish tank in the waiting area. There was a treatment room on the left side, with three entrances. Reclining chairs lined one wall and four hospital beds the other. Everywhere there were IV poles and pumps made by the brand Patient Pal. Ironic, don't you think?

The clinic atmosphere was fun. My primary nurse was Lisa Patrick, whom other patients nicknamed Pocahontas because of her Native American background. She was, of all the people in this strange new world, these new friends of mine, my favorite. She enjoyed teasing me for being quiet and always greeting her with a dull "hey" in my deepest voice. She called me a wuss if I winced when she drew my blood. I don't wince anymore.

The attitude of the staff towards the patients was informal—not what you'd expect considering how fucked-up the patients were. They were pale and completely hairless. They were people that I wanted nothing to do with, not because they were any different than me, but because I never thought I would be a Sick Kid. The reality was difficult to deny

in a room full of teenagers whom I would soon resemble. I was a Sick Kid. In the eyes of other people, I would never be able to discard the Sick Kid label.

Most of the patients on the floor were children, but two were in their twenties: Charlie Fletcher and Matt Cole. Charlie had been in the Army stationed in South Carolina and Matt was a mechanic for the Army in Georgia. They both had had to leave everything they knew in life to get treatment, at NIH. Funny, how cancer can end your life, yet the treatment to survive cancer also stymies your life progression, changing the tempo you had set for yourself. Your old goals become obsolete as nearly everything takes a backseat until you become healthy again. I was lucky, living nearby, that I could get home at night in an hour by crossing the Potomac River. There was a girl my age in the clinic, who also lived nearby. She remarked the day we met on how good-looking I was, which made me wonder if those days were over. Her name was Alexis Ernst. I didn't want to look like her, act like her or be sad like her, so I vowed to avoid her. I didn't want to have anything to do with other Sick Kids. However, I did know that, according to cancer, it was inevitable that I would have to.

So three days later, I climbed on the table in front of the cylindrical CT scanner. That three-minute scan of my lungs would reveal the probability of my survival. No spot, I would probably live. A spot and I would probably die. Simple statistical probability. That's how my parents and close relatives saw it. Me, I didn't even know what a CT scan was. I just held my breath as the robotic voice told me what to do.

The CT scan was just one of the eighteen tests I underwent the week before treatment began—measuring everything except the size of my dick. Alexis warned that it would be one of the worst weeks of my life, even calling it "Hell Week." There were two reasons for all those tests. The first was to make sure I was healthy enough for what was to come. The second was to create a baseline for the rest of my life.

The doctors expected that the functions they were measuring would worsen from the treatment, some of them immediately. I was only sixteen and already my health had climaxed.

Some of the tests were downright scary. One was an experimental procedure to try to create my own tumor vaccine. Theoretically, the vaccine leads to antitumor immune responses that can prevent tumor recurrence. To create the vaccine, the patient must undergo apheresis, a five-hour procedure where blood is withdrawn from one vein and a certain component is collected. The blood is then circulated back into the body through a vein in the other arm. The interesting thing about my tumor is that it didn't contain a specific protein found in most Ewing's sarcoma tumors.

Dr. Springs was uncertain whether the vaccine would even work. But I figured I would go through apheresis anyway, just to be on the safe side. How bad could it be? I would lie on this bed watching movies for five hours. But what if I have to piss? I asked the nurse as she stuck the IV in my left arm. "Don't worry about that, Ben. You can use a plastic urinal." She wrapped the tourniquet around my right arm and cleaned the spot with alcohol. I looked away as she pushed the needle through my skin and slid it up my vein. "Uh-oh," she said. Blood was streaming down my forearm.

My pulse sped up. My head pounded. I was sweating, dizzy and nauseous. I screamed at the nurse, "Take it out! Take it out!"

She called Dr. Springs down from Floor 13 to console me. He said, lying, that people often panic during apheresis. It was a kind gesture, but I didn't buy it. I turned into a nutcase because of some blood. If I couldn't handle apheresis, then how would I handle chemotherapy?

This time, my dad drove me home. I thought about death. I was drowning, alone and helpless. I sat in the back of his 1996 Chevrolet Astro minivan, or what I liked to call the Big Red Box, listening on my headphones to a mix CD Jonathan had burned for me. I heard what

immediately became one of my all-time favorite songs: Until We Rich, by Ice Cube & Krayzie Bone. I'll never forget them rapping, "The best thing in life is health."

Chemotherapy often affects the reproductive system. It can cause genetic changes to both sperm and egg cells, potentially causing birth defects. It can cause temporary or permanent impotence. More commonly it causes sterility. Dr. Springs advised me to freeze my sperm so it could be used later in life. I only had time to go to the sperm bank twice. Dr. Springs insisted I begin chemo as soon as possible while he knew it hadn't spread to my lungs. Killing the cancer was more important than the ability to spread my seed. Also, there was a no-ejaculation period of forty-eight hours before each visit.

My parents and I didn't have sex talks, and I learned most of that stuff from friends and David Duchovny's late-night soft-core series, *Red Shoe Diaries*. My dad knocked on my bedroom door the night before my first visit. "Hey Benjy, about the procedure tomorrow…do you know how to get it out? Do you need any help?"

"I know, Dad. No, I don't need help." This was about as awkward as when Drew had extreme diarrhea and the stall had been occupied. "I'm going to be in here for a while," the occupant had said. So, Drew had done what he had to: he dropped his pants, squatted, and crapped in the urinal.

My mom joined me on my first visit. We talked with the sperm bank director. "We have pornographic material for Ben to use if he'd like," he said. "Kill me now," I prayed.

"If he needs it," my mom said, thankfully not making me answer as she signed my consent form.

A cute nurse escorted me to my room. She showed me the magazines and told me to clean the tip of my penis with an alcohol swab. "Write how long it's been since your last ejaculation. Take as much time as you need. I'll be in the other room," she said. "Or you could stay and

help out for a while," I thought.

The room was small. It had a sink, a cabinet and a short brown couch. I tried not to count how many stains were on it. My task wasn't easy to complete, even with the help of *Gallery*. My mom was sitting in the other room knowing right at that moment I was jerking it, and cancer occupied my mind.

Old Benito wasn't cooperative, but he got the job done. I left the sample on the counter, and my mom and I left in silence. She dropped me off at school during lunchtime. I walked into the cafeteria and raised my arms in victory as my friends gave me a standing ovation.

Both of my parents joined me on my second trip to Fairfax Cryobank. "You already gave me permission to use porn. Is it necessary for you two to come this time?" I thought.

I was more relaxed and finished the procedure quickly. "Are you done already?" my dad asked.

I let my parents get a significant head start toward the Big Red Box, and I put on my headphones and cranked up the volume. None of us spoke about this again. My parents continue to pay a large sum of money to keep my sperm frozen, and I silently thank them for it.

Days later, we received a phone call regarding the results. My first sample was normal in volume but highly concentrated. My second sample had a high volume with a normal concentration of sperm. This Super Man had Supersperm.

Aside from worrying about sterility, I fantasized like a typical adolescent male, even once during a two-month hospital stint. My room had a large window. I would stare out, wishing to glimpse a girl in a miniskirt when the wind was blowing.

Many of my hospital days I thought about girls more than anything else, except for food. I would rank my nurses, both in total hotness, and in categories such as "nicest ass." One night I dreamt that my hottest nurse entered my room, took her clothes off and slid beneath the sheets with me.

TWICE

The dream was so real that I expected it. I prayed. God let me down.

Sometimes my nurses would enter my room at night while I was awake. When they turned around, I would quickly take a mental picture for later use. It's a shame there isn't a "Tivo for real life," because I would leave that on pause forever. I didn't want to get caught staring at their butts, so I captured quick glances. The pictures still did their job, though.

The human body has a way of taking care of business, whether you want to or not. For weeks I didn't want to. When I got my first wet dream, I knew something needed to be done.

At night the nurses don't knock because they don't want to wake the patient. Based on the meds schedule and the next blood pressure check, a young man can find the best opportunity to use those mental pictures. I prayed hard for my nurse to get naked, but I prayed even harder for her not to catch me jerking off.

From my two sperm bank samples, there should be enough semen to produce a few kids, should I choose to have a family. There is one catch: some cryobanks feel there's a time-frame for using frozen sperm. According to SpermBankDirectory.com, sperm may not be viable after being frozen for twelve years. It depends on how each individual's sperm reacts to the freezing process. By the time I'm twenty-nine, my boys may be useless.

My biological clock is ticking.

Tick-tock. Tick-tock.

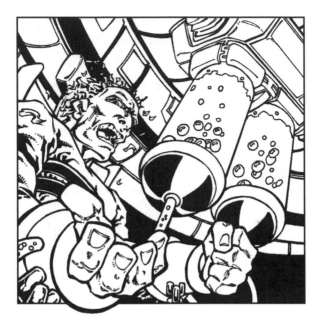

Chapter 2
THE TOXICITY IS WITHIN ME

Chemotherapy is poison. I had fourteen cycles of chemo; that sounds like a lot because it is a lot. Eight were long cycles consisting of five infusion days and six were short with only two days of chemo. Other than one long break between Cycles Five and Six, each cycle began three weeks after the previous one. I wished the Redskins' quarterback, Brad Johnson, could throw me two quick touchdowns so I would finish all fourteen cycles in a jiff.

The long cycle contained two chemo drugs and the short cycle was composed of three. Some of their side effects include: nausea, vomiting, hair loss, decreased red and white blood cell count, decreased platelet count, mouth sores, skin burns, anemia, weakness, sterility, weight loss, loss of appetite, loss of energy, tingling, pain, aching, constipation,

hoarseness, fluid retention, seizures, bladder irritation and bleeding, lung damage, liver damage, heart damage, kidney damage, sleepiness, confusion, the acquisition of a second cancer and death.

Mesna, which isn't chemo, protects the bladder from the toxic effects of the other drugs and is administered every four hours. If mesna was sent into my vein too fast, I would taste it. I would smell its stench in my urine. Before mesna became available in IV form, patients had to drink it. They said it was only tolerable if they mixed it with chocolate milk.

My friend Drew was fascinated by my pink-orange urine after receiving Adriamycin, the most toxic of all my chemotherapies. "Take a picture of your urine; I want to see it…after you have already pissed, of course."

Before each infusion of Adriamycin, I was given a drug to protect my heart, although it still has a maximum lifetime dose. A doctor once said to me, "You have already gotten a lifetime's worth of Adriamycin. Your heart can't take anymore. If your cancer comes back, we'll have to give you something else."

When I learned that I would receive a drug to protect my heart, I wondered what was going to protect my lungs, liver and kidneys. The answer: nothing. They inserted a port in my chest before my first dose of chemo. A port is a piece of plastic sewn into the upper pectoral muscle, beneath the skin. A tube then runs through the subclavian vein beneath the collarbone and stops at the heart. Ports are ideal for people receiving long-term medication, such as chemo. The fluid is sent straight to the heart, as opposed to the hassle of first traveling through a periphery vein. The port looked like a large bump on my chest and was proof that I had cancer.

The day of the insertion, Dr. Springs was waiting for me in the OR. "You have done this before, right?" I asked him. I fell asleep from the powerful anesthesia before he could respond.

A year later, after finishing treatment, my port was removed. That

was the last piece of physical evidence that confirmed I had cancer. I left the disease in the biohazard receptacle right alongside my port. I insisted the port be removed sooner than it normally was. Leaving it in is like purchasing health insurance, where you're betting on getting sick. I gave cancer recurrence a zero percent chance of happening. Besides, if my cancer did return, then having my port surgically implanted a second time would be the least of my worries.

Each day that went by without beginning chemo reduced my probability of survival, as if there were a percentage timer that continuously ticked down, ten-thousandths of a percent at a time. The teeter-totter of life levels off at the fifty percent mark, and then tips over to the other side until eventually there's a 500-pound wrestler named Yokozuna sitting across from you and you're dying.

One of the worst aspects of cancer is fearing what's next. Fearing the unknown. Once I had experienced each part of the routine, I was no longer scared. It was like having an injury that causes pain—once you're used to the pain, you learn to live with it, as long as it doesn't get worse. And when the pain does get worse, you get used to that and say the same thing. I suspect there's a pain threshold that acts as a breaking point.

I trusted my nurses to give me the correct drugs and dosages just as I trusted my parents to make the best hospital choice. It was my parents who constantly checked the bags of chemo to make sure all the information was correct. I was laid-back before treatment and I was going to stay that way. Cancer wasn't going to change that about me.

My first day of chemo was a piece of cake. My anti-nausea drugs knocked me out. After I woke up, my chemo was completed, and I watched television and then went to sleep so the next day could begin.

In the hospital, I had roommates come and go, and I tried to ignore them all. You're sick, I'm not. Your life sucks, mine doesn't. Just because we both have cancer doesn't mean we have anything else in common, I would think to myself. I wonder if subconsciously I did see myself as

sick. Maybe I even still do, but I expect that thought will stay buried for a long time.

My room was small with one bathroom and my bed was separated from my roommate's by a blue curtain. We each had a tiny television that we could rotate around our beds, although the only stations available were local networks and the hospital movie channel. The lack of ESPN should have been a human rights violation. The playroom had a select number of TV/VCRs, and my parents always snagged one if it was available. I watched my favorite comedies without asking my roommate's movie preferences. Anybody who doesn't like *Happy Gilmore* should be forced to drink mesna.

Opposite each of our beds was a small cot. One of my parents stayed with me every night I was there; just about every second, in fact. They probably thought that I always wanted or needed them there, but they were wrong. They annoyed me by waking me up, pulling on my IV line, investigating my bags of medicine and asking me questions. They responded to doctors and nurses for me, not by my request. They were chatty with all the patients, even the ones I wanted nothing to do with.

My frame of mind was different around my parents than it was around anyone else. I wondered, "Why can't you give me some space, preferably the same amount as you gave me before cancer, which wasn't enough to begin with? I'm still a teenager with a desire to act like one—do what I want, try to look cool, and fantasize about girls in private."

My parents' presence inhibited me from fully experiencing cancer as a patient. They smothered me. I brought part of that on myself with my clinging personality. You know the shy child who stays close to his parents when he's anxious? That was me long after I stopped being a child. My parents were always more restrictive with me than with Jonathan, and even with the freedoms of being sixteen, I still lingered around my parents, unlike most guys my age.

One of my nurses was an Orthodox Jew. She brought a chicken

dinner to my parents on Rosh Hashanah, the Jewish New Year. Rosh Hashanah occurs around the same time every year, when the leaves change, the nights darken and football begins. This was the season I began and, one year later, finished treatment. Rosh Hashanah now acts as a new beginning for me, a new year of cancer freedom, that sweet taste of apples and honey, that beautiful blow from the shofar giving me goose bumps and a grin that won't wipe away.

But that year, Rosh Hashanah represented not a beginning, but rather my lost year, devoid of honey. When my dad asked if I wanted to attend Rosh Hashanah services at the hospital chapel, I told him I didn't feel like it. God would cut me slack this time.

My dad is far more religious than I am. We always do the Passover Seder with his sister, my Aunt Florence. At the end of the evening, after dessert and when we're ready to go home, Aunt Florence and my dad always sing a few songs that seem to have no endings. When they were young in an Orthodox family, they would stay up the entire night praying with their relatives. My uncle tries to get away from the table by claiming he has a cold or pretending to be tired. It never works. And my dad and Aunt Florence have the most terrible singing voices. I would consider drinking mesna straight up than listen to their rendition of "Chad Gadya" ("One Little Goat".)

Later that night I called Drew to share my relief that chemo wasn't all that terrible. Drew was just living his normal life and I was living what had become mine. Getting out of the gossip loop was inevitable, considering I missed so many days of school. Andy got a new girlfriend, and I didn't meet her for a month. I didn't hold my friends back. I never said, "I'm not feeling well, come over to my house," or, "I just need someone to talk to."

No matter how cheerful I sounded, simply mentioning the subject of my troubles was an act of complaining to me. That's a standard I continue to keep. Looking back, I may have been fooling myself into

thinking that certain normal human emotions didn't apply to me. I don't know that my never mentioning cancer allowed others to misinterpret how sick I was. I never shared what my days were like, how important certain events were, or the cancer itself. But certainly that strong, silent outlook aided in my feeling of invincibility. All those other cancer patients complained about how hard it was, but I never once bitched.

The Saturday I was discharged from the hospital, I woke up and felt moderate pain in the area of my tumor. Instead of concentrating on how much they hurt, I experienced the pain as the sensation of the cancer cells dying. I told them, "Screw you, ass wipes. I am the ruthless destroyer of evil. You thought you could survive? I killed you in less than three days."

When I got home, I was falling behind in my classes. I couldn't focus. Even a vocabulary worksheet was hopeless. I could only think about cancer and how my life a few weeks earlier had been so much better than my life now. What a difference one cancer day can have on your spirits.

My friend Tim later asked me, "Why didn't you just quit school in your junior year when you got cancer? If I had been faced with that scenario, I think I'd quit."

"I was a top student my whole life. I wouldn't even know how to quit." I told him.

School rules were that I was either a regular student or I was home-schooled. I wasn't supposed to alternate between attending classes and studying at home, but nobody in the school administration wanted to mess with my mom. A few years earlier, my mom was sickened by discrimination in our area and co-founded the organization, "Unity in the Community," which tried to fight prejudice. When I refused to sing "Silent Night" while caroling in the fourth grade, my teacher put me in timeout. Funny how, after my mother got her organization going, that teacher never messed with me again.

My mom arranged for me to receive home schooling from a sarcastic young teacher named Mrs. Schumacher, or Shoomy as I liked to call her.

She taught Humanities at my high school. We met either in her class-room after school or at my house. On the days I did go to school I had freedom to do whatever I wanted, including sleep. One afternoon, I said to Drew, "I'll probably take a nap, so can you wake me up at 1:45? My mom is picking me up to go to NIH."

I fell asleep and Drew did what I asked. Our teacher, without know-ing I had asked Drew to wake me up, yelled at him. "Ben needs his sleep! Leave him alone!"

I dropped my two Advanced Placement classes, history and English, and took their remedial counterparts. The only difficult classes I had left were chemistry and functions analytic geometry, neither of which Shoomy knew anything about. My chemistry teacher didn't give a dead-line for when I had to turn in my homework and tests, so I snatched my friend's graded work and earned the easiest A of my life.

I ended my junior year with straight As, thanks to cheating and light-ening the workload; all of my classes except math were condensed tre-mendously. "Milk cancer for all it's worth," my enterprising friend Andy advised me.

Despite the good grades, not exercising my mind made me slack and stupid. Chemo brain symptoms like fogginess and problems with memory, word retrieval, concentration and processing numbers slowed me down for a while. My SAT scores declined significantly from the beginning and end of treatment. My intelligence has since returned close to its pre-cancer level.

I learned that limiting stress could do wonders for my mental health, just as I knew it could for my physical fitness. That whole year I tried to remain cool and relaxed. I felt that cheating and taking the easy path were vital to my well-being. They helped keep me stress-free, which gave me the best chance to survive. My parents knew about my cheating habits, but they looked the other way because they understood the con-nection between anxiety and health. They were willing to do anything

for me, including little cheats to reduce my stress. After cancer, my mom stopped bothering me about my homework.

Sunday was one occasion when I couldn't relax no matter what. My mom, after seeing me struggle with the vocabulary sheet I was working on, proposed that we go to Fuddruckers for lunch. I ordered the usual: one-third pound hamburger, medium-well, a side of fries, and a strawberry milkshake. My burger didn't taste like it usually did. Dr. Springs had told me that chemo might change my taste buds, and nothing I ate for the next year was going to taste the same.

I ate almost nothing. I knew that it takes a few days for chemo to completely exit a person's body but even so, on the ride home I became depressed. Reality finally hit me. School being more stressful was no big deal, but taking away food, one of my passions, made me miserable.

I doubted my ability to withstand the coming year. The idea that the cancer would spread throughout my body and kill me had never crossed my mind. For some people, the tumor doesn't respond well to the drugs, but I knew that my tumor would die from the chemo. It was probably already dead. Even so, on the ride home from Fuddruckers, I thought about killing myself for the first time. I didn't get into the details of when or how. I didn't consider whether my parting words would be funny or poetic. I just knew cancer had turned my life into something I did not like, and I wanted my old life back.

So when I got home, I called my friend Worm to come over and watch the Redskins game. Worm has been my friend all my life. I was the one who liberated him from his given name, Ethan Worman, to the cool "Worm." He is a huge Skins fan. But before the game even started, I got nauseous and rushed to the bathroom to puke. It looked like gallons of pink chunks, with some hamburger on the side. "Are you done yet?" Worm yelled. "That was disgusting. I could hear you all the way down the hall!"

The vomit was my emotional release. Once I barfed, my mood went from suicidal to giddy. Maybe cancer wasn't so tough after all. I went

back to my room to watch the Skins game with Worm.

The game went into overtime, when none other than "Prime Time" himself, Deion Sanders, returned a punt fifty-seven yards to set up a game-winning field goal. The Buccaneers had beaten the Redskins in the playoffs the previous season by one point. A bad snap on a field goal attempt at the end cost the Redskins a trip to the NFC Championship. Dan Turk was the snapper on that play, and he later died from testicular cancer. I blamed Dan for the loss.

From Worm that afternoon, I learned there were some things that not even cancer could change—my friends, my sense of humor and my love for the Redskins, to name a few. "I can do this," I said to myself. " One cycle down, thirteen to go."

It was good that I got a hold of myself because the next week some of my hair began popping out. I knew it was just a matter of time before I lost all of it. My curly hair is caused by each strand being misshapen and too flat. The imperfect strands clung to my pillow, stayed in the shower drain, or stuck between the keys of the piano.

I hoped getting my hair cut short would reduce the weirdness when it fell out completely. Worm agreed to get his hair cut with me. On the way, I popped two Ativans. "What are those?" he said.

"Anti-anxiety pills. I'm scared of getting a haircut and this may help."

I had always kept my hair short until the summer before my freshman year of high school. I didn't know if my hair would be wavy or curly, but as it turns out, it was really curly. I kept it well-groomed that year, but as a sophomore, I got only one cut and allowed my hair to take on a life of its own. I washed it twice a day with Pantene Pro-V shampoo, or some girly crap like that. Instead of a big curly ball of hair, I had long corkscrew locks that formed naturally.

The girls at my school wanted to play with it, including Andrea Buchman from my biology class, who wrote in my yearbook, "It's been

a great year. My favorite part is when I get to come in class to play with your wonderful hair. I swear I'm in love with it. I love you too, so don't get jealous. Have a good summer!"

Andrea wrote down her phone number. If I had not been such a pussy I would have called her. Other people were envious, including Worm, who wrote in my yearbook, "Get a haircut!" My hair was over eight inches long and stretched down to my chin. When I played tennis I wore a headband to keep it out of my eyes. I was going for the John McEnroe look, minus the mullet. Now I asked the barber to cut it as short as possible. He took the trimmer and buzzed away. I looked in the mirror and was frightened. "That's not me," I thought.

Worm and I went to the mall where I purchased a black Virginia Tech fitted hat to cover it up. During Jonathan's sophomore year at Tech, I had loved Michael Vick and the rest of the football team. The Hokies had an awesome season that year, going 11-0 until finally losing to Florida State in the National Championship.

I hated my buzz cut as much as Vick hated pit bulls. I began to wear a fitted baseball cap to hide my shaved head. I wore it everywhere until late November. Students weren't allowed to wear hats in school, but I got special permission.

One of my favorite teachers stopped me in the hall and told me to take my hat off. He didn't believe me when I told him that I had permission. Then I showed him my signed note from the assistant principal. When I walked away and adjusted my hat, fitting it tighter around my small head, I wished I could hide my whole body under it.

Worm said he would shave his head in my honor. "I'm going to wait until class pictures are finished because I don't want to be bald in the yearbook," he explained to me. "I am definitely shaving my head." It was a kind gesture but he got cold feet. I avoided all cameras that year. I wasn't even photographed for the yearbook. Someone took a Polaroid of me with those therapy dogs people bring to hospitals. I ripped it in half.

For a long time after the haircut I was scared to look in the mirror, scared of my own shadow. I would avoid looking at walls so I didn't have to see my silhouette. I preferred bathrooms with bad lighting. How could others recognize me when I can't recognize myself?

The first day I went to school wearing my Tech hat, my peppy friend Terry Pease said, "You're so lucky. You get to wear a hat to school every day!" "Yeah," I thought. "I'm real lucky, Terry. It's such a joy being allowed to wear a hat in school that I faked cancer just so I could wear it."

My hair started falling out in a serious way. I was reading on the floor one day when I felt an itch at the back of my head. After scratching, I brought my hand down to my book and was horrified—hundreds of tiny hairs engulfed my hand. I wiped them on the carpet and rubbed my head. Again, hundreds of hairs. They were detaching from my skull like foliage on a windy autumn day. I placed my head under the bath faucet. Apparently the hair really liked my hand, so I rubbed my head back and forth under the water, peeling off clumps with each swipe. Did all of these suckers decide to let go of my head at the exact same time? When I finished, I was nearly hairless, with a few patches toward the back and an irritated scalp. The rest of the hair fell out over the next day. I was as cancer-looking as it gets.

But it didn't look bad and even evoked some compliments. When Shoomy came for the first lesson after the chemo, she commented, "You have a nicely shaped head."

"Yeah, sure."

"No, I'm serious. Some bald people have weird lumps on their head, but not you."

I liked to think of myself as a young Vin Diesel, only paler, shorter, scrawnier, less Italian and more Jewish. And with more potent sperm.

The car rides to NIH that autumn are permanently etched into my brain. I can visualize the signs and scenery down Interstate 66. I can feel

myself in the passenger seat, and the anticipation of chemo years later still makes my stomach turn. At the Capital Beltway fork, I would have preferred to take I-270 North instead of I-495 toward Bethesda. Maybe I could stop in Pennsylvania Dutch Country and live with the Amish.

Years later, after graduating college and moving out of my parents' house, I took I-66 to and from work. The sensation of cancer was striking, like the eight-year gap in time was vacuumed into a black hole. I felt like a lost boy staring out the window into my past. I felt a strong love for my mom, her hands always at ten and two, her thumb resting on the horn, as she drove me to NIH for the torture that would heal me.

After chemo, I needed something that would cause diarrhea. I had been supposed to take a pill called Colace, a stool softener that increases the amount of water the feces absorb in the gut. Colace is a small pill, but even it was too much for me. Back then I could barely swallow my tiny red multi-vitamin, and missed many of my Colace doses. As a result, the only craps I had taken over the last week consisted of small, hard balls, which I referred to as nuggets.

When I arrived at NIH, the lunch lady was taking down orders and I chose SpaghettiOs. "You shouldn't eat those SpaghettiOs," another patient, Charlie, said. "That tomato sauce is brutal."

"He's right," Matt added. "You better be aware of your bowel condition. Sometimes, I have to crap so bad that I'm running to the bathroom every five seconds. Other times, I'm afraid to go because it feels like I'm shitting a brick."

Our bowel conditions represented our relative health. We may have had massive tumors, and our white blood cells may have been close to zero, but if our constipation was under control then we were perfectly fine.

I saw Christine Pinot, my nurse practitioner and medical guardian, on every visit. During her examination, she would listen to my belly. If it wasn't making sounds, she would say, "I think you might be constipated."

You think? Is it bad to not poop for a week? To help push things

through, Christine ordered me milk of magnesia from the pharmacy. I went to the waiting room and sat.

I still wasn't shitting, but I sure felt like shit. Aunt Florence had come to visit me and was ready to get food. "No thanks. I don't want anything," I said. "I'm just going to sit here."

"Of course I don't want food," I thought. "Look at me. I am waiting for the milk of magnesia to do its magic."

Aunt Florence is as difficult to sway as she is persuasive, but in this case she cooperated. She had brought me reading material, but I was afraid to move my arm to turn the page. My mom and aunt sat at the table with me, each reading her own book, like a dog owner patiently waiting for her poodle to poop.

You could have set a watch to my stomach cramps. As the minutes ticked away, they got worse. The first few times I tried pooping I had no results. When I left the bathroom, my aunt and mom stared at me with a "How did you do?" look on their faces, like I was three years old and learning to go potty. I shook my head and slouched back in my chair.

After several hours, I had a sharp abdominal pain, the worst yet. I rushed to the bathroom, swung the stall door open and flung the seat down. It was so painful I may have temporarily blacked out. I looked at my masterpiece. The whole scenario reminded me of the time my dad tutored a severely disabled little girl for her Bat Mitzvah. She took a long bathroom break in the middle of their session. When I went in later, I lifted the seat and saw a log stuck at the bottom of the toilet about the same size she was. My pile rivaled that one.

That night I switched to the liquid form of Colace, which is probably second in flavor to mesna. I drank it up to four times a day. In order to prepare myself, I composed a short jingle:

> Time for me to drink my Colace, it tastes so good.
> I have gotta drink my Colace, I bet you wish you could!

Coming to a radio near you! That nastiness of liquid Colace was not enough to tame the beast, so I added mineral oil twice a day. The grossest thing about mineral oil was the end result—I shat out the oil intact.

Even more important than our feces was our blood. A cancer patient's world revolves around blood counts. Different diseases focus on different analyses, but there are some that are critical no matter what you have. The most important blood test is the complete blood count, which gives the numerical value of different kinds of cells per unit of blood. White blood cells are the body's infection fighters. There are five types of white blood cells, including the neutrophil, which accounts for half of all white cells. Neutrophils are the soldiers of the immune system. Their job is to destroy infectious particles in the body. The absolute neutrophil count, or ANC, is the value doctors pay most attention to. A normal ANC value lies between 2,500 and 6,000 neutrophils/mm^3. When you have 1,000 or fewer neutrophils, you have an increased risk of infections. When the ANC drops below 500, you run a risk of getting a serious, possibly fatal, infection. This is called neutropenia. At this stage, your body no longer has the ability to protect you.

When you become neutropenic you must take every precaution to avoid infection: checking your temperature, washing your hands, staying away from people. This is an aspect of the cancer world that most people don't know about. Neutropenia is no joke.

The hemoglobin level is the second most important figure in the complete blood count. Hemoglobin is contained in red blood cells. It provides the lungs and tissue with the necessary oxygen needed to function. Normal hemoglobin values fall between 11 and 15 gm/dL. When your hemoglobin drops below eleven, you become anemic. When you're anemic, you may struggle to do even the simplest physical tasks, including standing up. This is because the body has less oxygen to work with. Anemic people constantly feel tired.

I stayed home from school because I was neutropenic. I watched

Big Daddy while my mom made me macaroni and cheese for lunch. It was one of my new staples, thanks to food restrictions during neutropenia. I barely ate; when I get depressed, I lose my appetite.

My sole reason for continuing to exist at this time was to wait for my white blood cells to rise. Another unproductive day ticked away. It didn't take long for me to see the benefit in this. Now I often judge my days based on how productive I am, whether it be exercising, engaging in social events, finishing tasks or doing work. When I had cancer, I could watch television the entire day and still I would consider myself productive. When, by the middle of the afternoon, I couldn't think of anything else to do, I watched *Big Daddy* again. I didn't consider my life was worthless because I watched the same movie twice in the same day. Instead, I felt I was delegating the task of producing the white cells to my body and waiting patiently while it did its work.

The next day, however, was different. It was Yom Kippur, the holiest day on the Jewish calendar, when Jews fast and pray. When I turned off the water from my shower that morning, I stepped over the tub and reached for my towel. The room began to spin. I glimpsed at myself in the mirror and my eyes rested on the disgusting bump in my chest. My figure was blurry, full of dark spots. I began shivering and became nauseous. My right ear started ringing, and I could hear my heartbeat. This must be death.

I assumed I was about to pass out, so I yanked on my boxers, scurried to my room, and sprawled out on my bed. I was experiencing acute symptoms of anemia, which had come on rapidly. Once I lay down, they went away. This was the tenth day of Cycle One, which my doctors warned me could be the worst. I would have appreciated it if they had informed me of the death symptoms.

All of my doctors had warned me about the seriousness of a fever while I was neutropenic. My parents were also obsessed with the possibility of a fever. They bought an ear thermometer to check my

temperature ten times a day. "Come on, Mom," I would have to tell her after she had checked my temperature three times in one morning. "I have a temperature of 100.3 and you're not allowed to take my temperature again for at least another hour," I would say. The threshold temperature that docs consider feverish is 100.4, so I would will my body to stay below that. This time, though, when the threshold was met, I was scared. I know what you're thinking: "But Ben, what's the worst that could happen? If you had a fever, why didn't you just wait it out like you were doing anyway?"

Aref, one of my favorite doctors at NIH, had told me: "Never take a fever lightly. Not long ago I had a young patient. She was neutropenic with a fever and her mom called, so I told her to get in the car and drive to NIH immediately. It took them a long time to get here. When she finally arrived it was four hours after her fever started and the infection had already spread across her whole body. She died later that day."

With this story resonating in my brain, I called out to my mom. I turned on the baseball playoff game between the New York Mets and San Francisco Giants while I frantically collected my things. I stuffed my bag faster than she packed hers, so I begged her to hurry. We had to drive to NIH, where I would be admitted until my ANC reached 500.

On the way there, I was tracking how long it had been since the thermometer displayed 100.4. My mom was driving slowly, but to me she couldn't drive fast enough. Never mind that a temperature of 100.4 is nowhere near dangerous, or that neutropenic fevers can be flukes that don't amount to actual infections, or that I felt physically fine. That was a fear I never, ever want to experience again.

We arrived to a calm hospital staff and not the frantic one I had expected. The nurse put me in a regular hospital room devoid of intensive care equipment. Nothing had to be resuscitated. Dr. Springs looked me over, noting the acne that had spread across my back was worse than J.J. Redick's.

After Dr. Springs left me, I switched on the baseball game that was now in extra innings, and I ate an entire grilled chicken sub, forgetting that I had no appetite. That day was a turning point in my treatment and understanding of cancer. It is necessary for doctors to implant fear in patients. But as I clarified what could and could not kill me—and why—I felt less like I was stricken with cancer, and more like I was surviving cancer.

Watching that game in the safety of the room at NIH made me realize everything was going to be okay. My parents were keeping an eye on my vital signs. The docs knew the numbers. They understood the risk. Despite my scary symptoms, I had gone back to my game knowing everything was going to be okay. I had been so terrified of neutropenia and the accompanying potential for death that I figured I would be too fucked-up to even watch the end of this baseball game. Instead, I saw Benny Agbayani crush a home run to catapult the Mets to a 3–2 victory. Who would have thought a simple baseball game between two teams I don't care about would have such a significant impact?

Sports were part of my regular routine. I watched all the baseball playoffs, every televised NFL game, and critiqued every Redskins game. The NFL kept my life moving. Each Sunday that passed meant that another cancer week was gone.

After a few hours, my dad came in to walk me down to radiology to get a chest X-ray. Every patient who was admitted for neutropenia received one as a precaution, along with vancomycin, an antibiotic. We got to talking about the Yankees, and how, even if you hate them, it's hard not to respect some of their players' postseason performances. Through 1999, Derek Jeter batted .326 in the playoffs. During that same time period, El Duque's ERA was 1.02 and Mariano Rivera's was a staggering 0.38 with thirteen saves. Rivera hadn't given up a single run in eighteen consecutive postseason appearances, including six World Series games. He may be the best postseason pitcher ever. It was sweet to have

something on my mind besides death.

Man, I needed something to hold on to during that first month of cancer treatment. With Jeter, El Duque and Rivera, the Yankees weren't going anywhere until they would beat the Mets in the World Series on October 26. I adopted the Yankees as my team, sharing them with my dad.

In the spring of 1958, the Brooklyn Dodgers had moved to Los Angeles, leaving my dad's Brooklyn family without a home team. The relocation didn't bother my dad much. His parents and Aunt Florence were never able to transfer their loyalties to the Yankees, but my dad, a rebellious thirteen-year-old, proudly wore his brand-new New York Yankees jacket to the dinner table. His family stared at him, horrified.

Forty years later, my family fell in line with my new-found love of the Yankees. Aunt Florence, whose jaw dropped at the dinner table so many years before, bought me a Yankees World Series hat. Jonathan bought me the red Yankees hat that Fred Durst—lead singer of Limp Bizkit—made famous.

Down at radiology, the technician instructed me what to do, but very soon it would be instinctual: remove shirt, turn to face white board and press chest against it, raise arms out to the sides, hold breath. Turn ninety degrees and raise arms above head, grab bar, press side against white board, hold breath.

Two days later, my white cells and hemoglobin began to increase. Since the effect chemo has on the body is cumulative, my bone marrow had not yet taken much punishment. I recovered quickly. Now there was nothing left Cycle One could throw my way: neutropenia was the last torture in a round of chemo.

A wave of unbridled happiness swept over me. My family stayed by my side and were stoked that I was in high spirits. I think I comforted all of them, the same way the playoff baseball game had comforted me the night before. To celebrate, my uncle brought me *Maxim*, eveb though I don't think my mom (who had reluctantly signed off on my

viewing porn at the sperm bank) ever intended for porn to become a habit with me. I would later trade the *Maxim* with Drew for the 2001 *Sports Illustrated* swimsuit issue, kind of like the way I used to trade my Gushers fruit snacks for Reese's Pieces at school lunch.

I was as soothed as if God sent an angel to whisper in my ear, "Benjamin, you are alive and that won't change on my watch." It was wrong for me to be so happy on Yom Kippur, the Day of Atonement, but I couldn't help it. I was high on life.

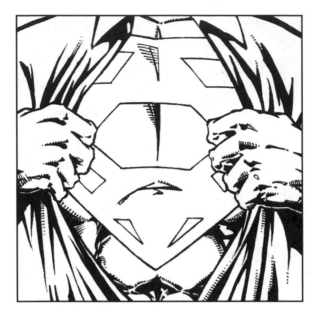

Chapter 3
BENJAMIN, HE-BRO PRINCE

At large treatment centers like NIH, patients are assigned a social worker to assist them and their families. My social worker, Ronne Schotter, took me into a private room to talk about the Make-A-Wish Foundation, an organization that grants wishes to any child between the ages of two and eighteen with a life-threatening illness.

"Can my wish be a car?"

I was imagining how many girls I would get if I drove a great car. How about a Batmobile? I would invite Lily for a ride home and show her my machine gun. "It has a shield and rocket launcher, too," I would tell her. "I see that it also has ejection seats," Lily would say. "But the only place we're going is downtown."

Ronne was looking at me trying to figure out how to answer. "I

don't think we can get you a car. But you can get a lawnmower. They won't get you anything that goes over ten miles per hour."

"I don't know, Ronne. I don't need anything. I think I'll pass and let someone who needs it get something."

The Make-A-Wish Foundation was designed to give children hope and inspiration. I wasn't a child and didn't need external motivation. If I did make a wish, it would be some activity or material object for my own pleasure.

When I had gotten home from the hospital after Cycle Two, I talked to my friend Andy about my wish. "I could try to get a guest spot on an episode of *Friends*."

"No way, this is what you should do…have them get you a hooker."

"I'm sure that would fly with my parents. You know they have to sign off on this."

"That doesn't matter. Tell them you need it for your cancer. Tell them to get a second hooker for me."

If there had been no restrictions, then I would have gotten the Batmobile. With the ability to reach 350 miles per hour with afterburner thrust, I would never be late to anything again. And I would always have a hot girl with me when I arrived. Other ideas included:

- Getting an acting role in a TV show.
- Taking a trip to Hawaii.
- Playing football at FedEx Field. I would ask Champ Bailey and LaVar Arrington to join me and my friends in a game of two-hand touch.
- Shooting hoops with Michael Jordan.
- Meeting President Clinton.
- Getting tickets to WrestleMania.
- Meeting Britney Spears or Christina Aguilera for the sole purpose of getting play. I was leaning toward Aguilera because I thought she'd be more likely to put out.

I narrowed my wish down to playing football with the Washington Redskins and going to Super Bowl XXXV in Tampa, Florida. Then I had my epiphany and I figured out what I really wanted: an entertainment system worthy of being on *MTV Cribs*. My parents got a letter in November saying the Foundation was honored to fulfill my wish. "It is our desire that a wish fulfilled will provide your son with hope, strength and joy as he fights his illness." I didn't know about all that, but I did know it would make my ass-sitting time much more pleasing.

In December, two representatives from Make-A-Wish Foundation arrived at my house with my new toys: a fifty-three inch Hitachi High Definition Digital Television, a five-speaker Sony surround sound system, a VCR and a DVD player. As if that wasn't enough, they later bought me a DirecTV satellite dish and an HD satellite receiver. The TV was bigger than the shelf, so my parents hired a carpenter to build a new platform. I was watching sports and Denise Richards movies in high definition before most people knew what HD was.

After our tutoring session one afternoon, I brought Shoomy down to the basement to see the system. "I think your TV is bigger than my living room!"she said.

"I know it is."

"Look at you, you're gloating. You showed me the TV just to brag, didn't you?"

"No, of course not."

"Why don't you open up the blinds to get some natural light in here?"

"The instructions for the TV say that you can't let sunlight hit it."

"You're such a dork."

"Don't hate it just because you're jealous."

And so I went on with my life as if nothing was wrong. It's just a little cancer, no big deal. My treatment followed a precise schedule: when the cycles begin, when they end, when to expect my ANC to drop, when I'll be neutropenic, and when my ANC will rise back to a safe level. For

Cycle One, I was admitted to NIH for neutropenia on Day Ten (ten days from the start of the cycle). Since Cycle Two was also a short cycle, I knew that on Day Ten, the same day as the Homecoming Dance, I would probably be hospitalized for neutropenia.

My cancer had increased my social status at school, so I was up to be one of the Homecoming Princes. I received nearly enough votes to win. In the past, I had gone relatively unnoticed, but now people were seeking me out to talk about sports. Everyone was overly nice to me, including friends who had always poked fun at me. I didn't want to be treated differently.

One week before the Homecoming Dance I was walking out of the lobby when my friend Terry called to me, "Have you asked anyone to Homecoming yet?"

"No."

"Would you maybe want to go with me?"

"I can't. I'm going to be sick that day and I won't be able to go."

I have known Terry since the seventh grade, where she was one of the few from my homeroom class whom I didn't invite to my Bar Mitzvah. She's been giving me a hard time about that ever since. I didn't invite her because she was so pretty and blond that she intimidated me. I couldn't bring myself to hand her the invitation.

Terry is also too tall for me but that's not the reason I turned her down for Homecoming. I shouldn't have been so blunt. How was she supposed to know what I meant by "I'm going to be sick that day"—who talks like that? Who can know in advance when they are going to be sick?

But true to my prediction, I woke up the morning of the Homecoming Dance—the tenth day of Cycle Two—unable to move without becoming light-headed. I had terrible mouth sores, called mucositis. Mouth sores are a common side effect of chemo and occur from a breakdown of the tissue lining the mouth (chemo targets rapidly dividing cells like those in cancer, hair, blood and the intestinal tract). Because I was

neutropenic my body couldn't repair the sores until my white blood cells increased.

By late morning my temperature reached 100.5, so my mom drove me to NIH. I could barely walk to the elevator. When reminiscing about the experience, my mom said, "I thought I was going to have to drop everything to catch you, you were about to collapse. Once we reached Floor 13, you had to sit down because you were shaking like a leaf. I ran to the nurse's station. They brought you a wheelchair, got you into bed, and gave you a warm blanket."

I almost always refused the wheelchair. I believe that if I can stand, then I can walk. Most people would call my condition "being sick." I called it, "fucked-up." Even years later, my friends make references to when I was sick. I correct them. "Don't you mean when I was 'fucked-up?'"

"Fucked-up" made me feel strong. I didn't see myself as sick because I was just a normal person who happened to be receiving deadly poisonous drugs to fight off the round cells that were attacking my body. When I told Terry, "I'm going to be sick that day," I broke my own rule. Terry thought that I didn't want to go to the dance with her, and that I used cancer as an excuse to reject her.

My friends teased me about that short conversation for the next two years. I thought, "If you only knew what I went through! You guys think I was chilling at my house watching my new HDTV and eating popcorn while you were at the Homecoming Dance?"

While I watched college football on the tiny TV back at NIH that night, I became hungry and sent my mom down to the cafeteria to get me a hamburger. I ate half. Each bite was excruciating; the two sores on the side of my mouth and the one under my tongue inhibited my eating, drinking and talking. With my neutrophil count of two, the sores weren't going to heal anytime soon.

As idiotic as it sounds, I thought my ANC was the total number of neutrophils swimming around my veins. When I was told my ANC was

two, I said, "How do they know I have two neutrophils in my body from just a small blood sample?"

My nurse explained. "That means you have two neutrophils per cubic millimeter of blood."

Dr. Springs found a solution to my mouth pain. "I have a topical anesthetic called lidocaine viscous that might do the trick," he said. "I tried it out earlier to make sure it works. I didn't read the instructions and swished it around my mouth. You're supposed to dab a Q-tip in the bottle and paint it on the sores."

"What happened?"

"Well I can't feel my mouth right now, but it definitely worked."

Dr. Springs chuckled. Like all the NIH Fellows, he switched between stints at NIH and Johns Hopkins. He and Aref, who didn't want to hear the "Dr." title beside his name, were the only ones who seemed human.

The Redskins played the Tennessee Titans on Monday Night Football the following night. The game was a big deal at the hospital, with some of the nurses understandably slower in their duties while sneaking peaks at our tiny TVs. The Redskins beat themselves with sloppy play and lost 27-21, snapping a five-game winning streak.

When I was discharged, I was excited to go home. I had gone trick-or-treating every year of my life and wasn't about to miss it now because of a petty problem like cancer. Most of my friends gave up trick-or-treating in high school in favor of parties. Like many traditions, especially those revolving around holidays, I couldn't let go, no matter what my age was.

In the eighth grade, I trick-or-treated in two neighborhoods with two different groups of people, steadfast in my wish for a long, continuous sugar high. Unlike Jonathan, who devoured his candy (he once ate fifty Starburst in eight minutes), I was a saver. I ate my final Snickers well into the winter. My candy would have lasted until the summer if Jonathan hadn't stolen some. I should have made him eat the Almond Joys for punishment. Or drink mesna.

I wore my Undertaker mask as I had the previous three years. Prior to cancer, I couldn't wait to take off the mask because it made me sweat. But all this year, looking like a Sick Kid had made me wish I had a mask to hide my face the way my caps hid my bald head. On that Halloween night, behind Undertaker, I felt like the old Benjamin for a brief few hours. But then it was back to NIH for the re-staging scans to see what my tumor had been up to. It had shrunk substantially, proving the chemo was doing its job. I expected nothing less. It was my tumor, and I had never lost a battle yet. Unfortunately, not everybody's tumor shrinks, but I knew that mine would. I had trouble understanding how some people could receive chemo that didn't kill their tumors.

I also struggled with the idea that not everybody expects perfect results. In a lot of cancer books, you read about acceptance of the disease, and death, too. Do they actually acknowledge the possibility that the cancer might kill them? I realize now that by not fearing my demise, I missed out on something special, something unique to survivors, a feeling that cannot be manufactured. These survivors say they felt like they could do anything, that the world was in their grasp. They say their fears were wiped away, like their fear of rejection or saying something stupid. They could live in the moment, care-free, having already faced death, having nothing to lose.

Short cycles are awful, but how are long cycles? Since my cancer friends had all begun treatment before me, I asked which cycle was more tolerable but got mixed reviews. The short cycle was relatively quick, and the long cycle was less harsh on our bone marrows. There was nothing fancy about the long cycle: five consecutive days of two chemos, one after the other, each taking exactly an hour to infuse. My chemo routine was long and grueling, with few deviations.

This sequence is repeated until I'm discharged.

Over the hospital stay, my hunger intensified. I felt a constant stomach

pain. "I'm going crazy," I said to Dr. Springs. "I keep seeing commercials for the new Pizza Hut Twisted Crust Pizza. Those perfectly seasoned breadsticks wrapped around the whole pizza, ready to be dipped. I can't stop thinking about it. I even dreamed about it."

"I figured all you thought about was girls."

"No, I think about the Redskins too." After two consecutive losses, the Redskins had gotten a needed bye but I was still watching football games on the itty-bitty TV. For the fourth consecutive day, I felt terrible, and eating made me feel worse. I kept throwing up. Even thinking about food could make me nauseous. None of the doctors at NIH worried about my nutrition. "You'll eat when you feel like it, no big deal." They believed that the chemo regimen was the only thing that killed the cancer: not your attitude, diet or God Himself.

My parents hated that NIH put little emphasis on diet, but I loved it. Since none of the doctors pressured me to eat, and eating didn't help me survive, I never felt guilty when I didn't. During Cycle Three, I went five consecutive days eating almost nothing, and my parents were the only ones who bothered me about it.

I decided not to eat until the cycle was finished. It was my rule—to punish myself during chemo by not eating, and reward myself with food at the end. That deprivation made normal eating unbelievably sweet. It made me appreciate the sense of taste more than ever before. Nowadays, I look forward to fasting on Yom Kippur, in hopes I can regain that appreciation. But it's just not the same as those long days of the chemo cycles.

The morning after the last day of chemo, I woke up ready to go home, but my hemoglobin had dropped under eight and I needed a blood transfusion. A blood transfusion consisted of two units of blood, each in its own bag, each bag taking two hours to infuse. I took Benadryl and Tylenol to prevent a reaction or fever, in which case the transfusion would halt and the blood would be discarded.

Before I started cancer treatment, my mom read an article claiming

that the American Red Cross failed to screen some blood. She wouldn't allow me to receive any stranger's blood, but instead had volunteers drive all the way to Bethesda to donate. Statistics show that direct donations are no safer.

Blood donations have a forty-two day shelf life, after which they are discarded. Direct donations—drawn for a specific person—could not be used for anybody else. My mom claims to have planned the donations perfectly, but it was impossible to predict exactly when I would need a transfusion. My homeroom teacher, Mr. Foley, claims that I'm one-third his because I have gotten so much of his blood. Maybe if I got Tom Brady's blood, I would be playing quarterback for the Patriots and marrying a Brazilian supermodel.

The bag was dark red with a large A+ written on the front. I was hooked-up to tubing, just as I had been for chemo, with two IV lines; one connected to the blood bag, and the other to a small bag of saline. If I reacted, the nurse would close the blood line, and the saline would begin immediately.

I watched as the thick red liquid slowly crept its way down the tube. Once out of sight, I lifted my shirt and stared as it entered the giant needle in my chest. I wanted to know the exact second it hit my bloodstream.

I watched *Billy Madison* followed by *Liar Liar,* and then *Dumb & Dumber.* Each bag took longer than two hours, so it was six o'clock by the time I was discharged. My nurse pulled the huge needle out of my chest and covered the bleeding hole with a Band-Aid. I darted out of bed and rushed my mom out the door. The blood gave me an extra boost of energy, like a vampire. I was furious that I had to stay there so late, my quadriceps were weak from disuse and I was famished. "Let's get out of here and go to McDonald's," I thought.

My mom thought it was an awful idea for me to eat greasy McDonald's so soon after receiving chemo, but I insisted. The ride home was just over an hour. It felt like eternity. I could see nuggets and fries,

and sundaes, oh my. My mouth watered with the thought of a succulent burger. We passed two McDonald's en route to my favorite one.

I shouted at the drive-through speaker, "I'll have the Double Quarter Pounder with cheese value meal, with a Coke. No mustard." I had never eaten a double QPC, but there was no better time to try than now. I demolished the fries by the time we got home and then ate most of the burger. I didn't vomit or get nauseous. If this had been a short cycle, I would have thrown up a kidney.

On the days leading up to Day Ten, I felt great, but I still expected to become neutropenic. However, my ANC didn't drop below 1,000. I received two potent chemos, and my immune system stayed normal, as if it was barely affected. Even though I had two entire weeks of freedom, in my opinion the long cycle was still worse. Those five days were that bad.

I once said to the nurse, "Have you noticed that I haven't been neutropenic for a long cycle, yet?"

"Yeah, Ben, that's really amazing."

"Have you ever seen that before? Everybody else seems to get neutropenic after long cycles."

"No, I can't recall that happening. Some people, like Alexis, get neutropenic but don't get a fever. That's pretty common for the long cycle."

Along with Supersperm, I had Super bone marrow. Several months later, when another patient finished treatment, he headed back home to Florida. When I said good-bye to him, he gave me a gift. "I saw this in the store, and I was thinking of you," he said as he handed me Superman boxers and a blue Superman t-shirt. Now my Super-Jew shirt has something to play with. "You have earned it," he said.

I was flattered that my fellow cancer patients noticed my powerful super marrow and recognized it was superior to anyone else's. Alexis always joked about how easy treatment was for me compared to everyone else. "You breeze right through this stuff," she said.

I saw my resilient bone marrow as a sign that I was supremely capable of battling cancer. I had something extremely unique, and I reveled in it, almost to the point of wanting to see others suffer just to fuel my ego. I was better than the other patients, better than everyone, better than humankind. I was The One. I was a Super Man.

However, my parents were definitely not Ma and Pa Kent, who had the tact to disappear when Clark was in high school. "You and dad act like I'm going to die and it pisses me off. I'm not going anywhere," I told them.

"We don't act like that," my mom responded. "What are you talking about?"

"Every day you guys ask me how I'm feeling, or if I need anything. You treat me different than you did before the cancer. I feel perfectly normal. Just cut that shit out."

"Oh, Benjamin!"

Much more often than before the cancer, my parents told me "I love you," and tried to touch or kiss me like I was two years old. "Get off me," I wanted to say, but held back. Once my mom didn't eat the last of the soy ice cream because she thought I might want it. I snapped at her. "Why the hell would I care if you eat it or not?" As soon as the words were out of my mouth, I wondered what kind of monster I had become. Why couldn't I accept signs of love? My parents loved me too much, and sometimes I wished they cared less. Even today, I recoil when I am shown acts of kindness or when others try to touch me.

Whenever my dad would arrive home from work, we'd have the same conversation:

"Hey Benjy, how are you feeling today?"

"Fine."

"Good. And how are you doing?"

"Good."

I answered the same way even if I felt awful. Eventually I changed

our conversation, which we carry on to this day as a joke:

"Hey Benjy, how are you feeling today?"

"How you feelin'?"

"I'm good, but I was asking you. How are you doing?"

"How you doin'?"

"Well I'm fine, but how about you?"

"How about you?"

Answering truthfully only gave Dad incentive to continue worrying about me. No matter how I felt, I wanted to appear fine. Some people may have appreciated the extra attention, but I despised it.

On my next trip to NIH, the social worker asked if Mom and I could talk in a private room. "I know you have things under control, but your mom asked me to speak to the both of you."

"This is about me saying that my parents treat me like I'm dying, isn't it?" I turned to the social worker. "I can't stand the way Mom babies me. It's like she doesn't realize cancer is temporary. I'm the same as I was before it and the same as I will be when it's over. In the words of Forrest Gump, shit happens. My shit happens to be cancer."

"But, honey, it's only because I love you," my mom said.

"I know. Just keep that stuff to yourself."

"I'm going to talk to your dad and make sure he knows that you don't like the way he acts around you," the social worker said.

My dad talked to the social worker that time and many other times, for what seemed like hours. I didn't know what they talked about, nor did I want to. It angered me, not that he talked to her, but that he needed to. I wanted him to see that I was stronger than the other patients. I wanted him to know that his son was special. I was disappointed that he wasn't as strong as me. I could not feel the sadness for my parents' pain that I was supposed to feel. Instead, I felt sad that my father, who never would have spent time with a social worker or psychiatrist before my cancer, was now hanging on their every word. He seemed to be losing

his wonderful quirky edge. I had always been kind of proud that my dad was a little crazy.

On my thirteenth birthday, he had been bitten by a huge black dog during his morning walk and had carried a bat, stick or pipe ever since, always prepared to clobber threatening animals. That includes cats, squirrels or guinea pigs—my dad assumed they were all rabies-stricken carnivores. He always walked at a brisk pace, wearing a baseball cap and listening to his Walkman, waving a weapon as if he could take on any living creature. What was sad to me was seeing him transformed into a submissive client, following the directions of a social worker half his age to leave his psycho son alone.

Even though I was let down by my dad and annoyed by my mom, I still loved my family, especially as Thanksgiving rolled around. My mom's family is scattered across the country; her sister Elsa and her mother live near each other in suburbs of Chicago, and her brother lives in Plano, a suburb of Dallas. We usually had an annual family reunion in Illinois.

The year I was first diagnosed with cancer, I said to Mom, "If you ever want your family to celebrate Thanksgiving at your house, now is your chance." Mom loves having company. "If you use my cancer as an excuse, they'll hop a jet over here to Virginia." This was the only time I didn't scold my mom for profiting from my cancer. I guess I knew she was going through a lot and since I share her nostalgic personality, I could see that a family reunion at home would make her happy.

My mom wishes our family behaved the same way the ideal American family does. Part of her rubbed off on me. The Macy's Thanksgiving Day Parade is terribly boring, but I tune in for a little while every year because I'm supposed to. I couldn't admit that I wanted a big Thanksgiving with my relatives because that's a desire often expressed by women, so I let my mom make it happen for me.

My idea worked—there's no better way to get the family together than by pulling the cancer card. We packed the house with thirteen

people including my grandma, my aunt, my uncle and their families. When they arrived, I was wearing a beanie. Even though I didn't want my young cousins to remember me all their lives as the cousin with cancer, I finally took the beanie off. They admired my nicely-shaped head. I thought if I left my hat on they would forget I had cancer. But when I removed my beanie, nobody was freaked. Maybe they were playing it cool, but they seemed surprised by how relatively healthy I looked.

They had been hearing my mom's dramatic accounts of how sick I was, so they were expecting worse than they got. We didn't have caller ID back then, so whenever I answered the phone, I was risking that a relative would consume my time asking cancer questions. Jonathan urged me to find an excuse to get off the phone, but I could never do it. I actually began enjoying speaking with Aunt Elsa.

On Thanksgiving my cousins and I played walking football in the street, since I wasn't allowed to run. My parents stared through the screen door to make sure I wasn't running. "You two have lost your minds," I told them when we finished playing. They were still fussing over me, despite what the social worker had said, but I tried not to make a scene about it.

My mom and Aunt Elsa grew closer because of my cancer. Aunt Elsa later claimed that my mom talked about my cancer too much, and once I was well, there wasn't anything left to talk about, so they drifted apart again.

The week after Thanksgiving, I chose to receive chemo for Cycle Four as an outpatient. Aunt Florence handed my mom the key to her house in Northwest Washington and said, "Stay whenever you want, even if I'm not home. The key is yours." She and my uncle were gone most of the time, so usually it was just me, one of my parents, and their dog, Barney.

Doing Cycle Four as an outpatient worked well for me. Aunt

Florence had just installed a large flatscreen television in view from the couch, although it didn't compare to my fifty-three-inch sweetheart. I spent a lot of time on the PlayStation 2 that Aunt Florence had given me for Hanukah. PS2s were hard to come by, but my aunt's friend had a preorder ticket for the first batch which Aunt Florence had gotten for me by using her charm. One evening when Aunt Florence was home, she wanted to prepare dinner for me and my dad. "I'll cook anything you want," she offered.

"I don't care, but my dad probably wants salmon, so let's go with that."

My parents loved salmon and made it for dinner every week. I associated salmon with chemo, and later became nauseous just from its scent. I developed an aversion to other foods as well, including Uno's Pizza. It took me three years before I was able to eat Uno's again, but I guarantee nothing will ever get me to eat salmon—ever.

On Sunday the Redskins played the New York Giants. I have seen every Redskins game since 1997, so even though I received chemo during the game, I was determined to stay awake. At the treatment room I saw Aref talking to another patient who looked my age. He was sitting in a wheelchair with a bag of urine hanging from his side. The tube that led to the bag came from somewhere beneath his shirt, probably directly from his bladder. "When you're done here, do you want to go get a steak?" Aref asked the boy.

"Yeah, Aref, that would be great," the patient said.

I learned two important things from that encounter: (1) Aref is a great doctor and person. He cared about us, not just as his patients, but also as his friends. (2) Drink plenty of water. That boy's kidneys were likely damaged from the chemo, and he could no longer urinate on his own. I sat behind him and couldn't stop staring. I felt bad for him, which is a cardinal sin among people with life-threatening illnesses because we don't need pity. I also felt superior to him. I drank tons of water. The bathroom became my haven. I thought of urinating as my personal

attack on cancer, a perfect complement to chemo. The more I peed, the more I got rid of the toxins. This is a habit that will never go away.

I won't end up like him. My body is stronger than his. I wanted to believe that. I had to believe that.

The Redskins lost to the Giants 9-7. After a great season start, they lost four of five games, their only win coming two weeks earlier on Monday Night Football over the high-powered Rams. I stayed awake, although I couldn't recall many plays.

Today I wonder if that boy survived, and if so, what his quality of life is like. He was in a hell I have never known and seemed happy with his friend Aref. If I were in a wheelchair with a tube through my bladder, I would not be able to still see myself as superior. I might even pity myself. If that kid did survive his cancer, then he probably faced organ dysfunction. So many people are surviving cancer nowadays that there's a new line of research dedicated to the long-term complications that appear months to years after treatment, which are known as late effects. I exempted myself from these late effects the same way I had refused to consider dying from the cancer itself. For many people, surviving cancer is not the end. Chemo is so toxic that there is no end.

Cancer provides an abundance of time. So often cancer patients are incapacitated, unable to contribute to society or even to ourselves. We try to waste time, make it go faster. I listened to a lot of music. And when I had enough energy, like when I rode home from the hospital with my mom on those cold fall nights, I pondered. I considered the enormous change my life had taken in such a short time. I thought about how strange, almost surreal, it was that I actually had cancer. I contemplated how I had become an outcast, different from everyone in a way that's obvious just by looking. I wondered how others viewed me.

I thought about school, wondered if anything exciting had happened there and the funny things I missed, and what my friends were doing. I dreamt about Lily and every other hot girl at school, and wondered if any

wore tight pants or a thong that day, and if you could see the outline of their underwear. I thought about playing backyard football and how much I missed it. I thought about the Redskins and wondered if they'd miss the playoffs for the seventh time in the last eight years. I thought about how I loved the cold air, bare trees, and dark nights. It was so peaceful.

I wondered how much the chemo would screw me up in the next cycle and how low my blood counts would drop. I thought about how cool it would be if I had a stress fracture instead of bone cancer. I thought about my upcoming surgery.

I thought about the other cars on the road, all those red and white lights. Why were their drivers out tonight? Where were they were going, and where were they were coming from? I had cancer, and that's the reason I was on the road, but what were their stories? They were just a few feet away, yet I would never know. As a teenager, I always had to tell my parents where I was going and when I would be back. What would it be like to be able to go anywhere I wanted without telling anyone? In just four years, I would be an adult and able to do that. I thought about what it would be like to not be a teenager anymore. That night, those years between me and twenty-one seemed a lifetime away.

Over the next two weeks, I thought a lot about growing up. I knew I would have to grow up in a hurry because my surgery was only a month away. My surgeon, Dr. Merlin, was famous. He was one of the first to perform limb-sparing operations for tumors. I had first met Dr. Merlin and his right-hand man, Dr. Wodajo, two weeks before treatment began. "Has anyone told you that you look like Brian Mitchell?" I had asked Dr. Wodajo at that first meeting.

"Who's Brian Mitchell?"

"He used to return kicks for the Washington Redskins."

"I don't have time to watch sports."

"Well, you have probably seen him in the newspaper."

"I don't have time to read the newspaper either," Dr. Wodajo said

with a smile.

Dr. Merlin was old, with white hair and a white mustache. He always wore a suit and walked as if he had the biggest dick in the world. He never smiled, but he had a quality that made me feel good—I think it was his confidence, which seeped out of his pores and into his patients. It wasn't just that he thought he was all that and a bag of chips; he knew he was all that and a bag of chips.

Dr. Merlin was always surrounded by an entourage of other doctors when he visited patients. They didn't speak, but stood silently as they learned the tools of the trade from their master. At the meeting before my surgery, Dr. Merlin brought me down to earth with the facts of what was going to happen to me. I had been taking my treatment in stride, not thinking too far ahead. Now he alarmed me with the schedule: two weeks in the hospital, one week in traction, followed by a brace to keep my leg abducted and no weight-bearing for ten to twelve weeks. Then, major rehabilitation. Up until that meeting, I had been focusing on my survival and not on what was actually getting cut away from me. If I had thought about that, I would have soiled my pants. "There is one thing you can do for me between now and then," Dr. Merlin said. "I want you to gain ten pounds because you won't be able to eat for about a week after surgery."

"Me, gain ten pounds? I don't think that's possible."

"Go to McDonald's and eat Big Macs. Those will beef you up," Dr. Merlin said.

"Or have your mom buy you milkshakes," Dr. Wodajo suggested.

My mom was overjoyed. "We have already been getting him milkshakes. The ones they have at Baskin Robins have over 1,000 calories."

I waited the entire visit before asking him the most important question I had ever asked anyone. "Will I ever be able to play tackle football again? Because to me that means complete recovery."

"Absolutely," Dr. Merlin said. "You'll be playing football again in two

years, and should be completely normal in five." That's what he thinks. I knew I would be playing football long before two years. It was not going to take five years before I was completely healed.

When I got home, I took my bicycle out for a spin. I couldn't deny that my recovery would be lengthy, or that my rehab would be difficult. Just a couple of weeks earlier, I had bumped into Friedman at school, and he had asked if I was going to play tennis in the spring. "I hope so," I had said. "I'm having surgery in early January, and I don't know how long recovery will take. I think I'll be able to play, though...if not this year, then certainly next year."

I couldn't understand why recovery would take so long. My super powers prevented my comprehension because it would have brought me down to acknowledge my cancer surgery's disruption could be life-long. I thought I would get stuff cut out, stay off my leg so it could heal, do some exercises, and that would be it. I would be back on the tennis court in no time.

Why would I be in the hospital for two weeks? What was I going to do in a hospital for that length of time? What would happen if I didn't have surgery and left the bone in my body? I mean, the tumor's already dead, right? Plus, I'm still going to get ten more cycles, which would certainly kill all the cancer cells. During my bike ride, I saw Drew driving home. He pulled alongside me, rolling down his window. "What are you doing?" he said.

"Just riding. Anything exciting happen at school?"

"No, not really. How did your doctor thing go?"

"He said my hip wouldn't be back to normal for five years."

"Sorry man, that sucks. At least you'll have more time to play your PS2, you bastard."

My friends had started coming over all the time since I was the only one with PS2. When Andy arrived later that afternoon, I told him how I was supposed to gain ten pounds. "That's awesome," he said laughing.

"I know. How often does your doctor instruct you to eat the McDonald's Heart Attack Special?"

My mom lived up to her word and brought me a Baskin-Robins milkshake almost every day. You can get an idea of how big a deal this was only when you know that my parents, who both have elevated cholesterol, watch their diets closely. They do not eat ice cream and as far as I know, have never touched a Baskin-Robbins milkshake. When I was ten, I started getting annual cholesterol tests. I hated them, but the smiley face stickers I got after the pricks made them worthwhile.

When I was thirteen, I voluntarily went on a low-fat diet for one year because my cholesterol was high. The following summer my family went on vacation to Hershey Park. After riding through the chocolate factory, we were all given Hershey's Kisses. "I'm not allowed to eat these," I said as I handed them to my brother. An hour later I couldn't take it anymore and guzzled two pints of chocolate milk. One of cancer's gifts was my parents' new-found lack of concern over my fat and cholesterol intake. Not only were they willing to buy me high-fat foods, they actually took pleasure in it.

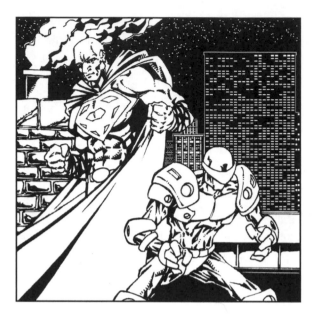

Chapter 4
DOWN FOR THE COUNT

Cycle Five was a piece of cake because Jonathan came home for winter break. He joined us at Aunt Florence's house. Up till then, he had been coming home to visit every three weeks, when my blood counts were high and I was relatively healthy. When he was at school, he had to rely on reports from my mother, who could make a cold sound like swine flu. We talked on the phone every afternoon, briefly touching on my cancer before we moved on to more important things, like how the Redskins were doing.

I was looking forward to having Jonathan around. Since this was the first time he had seen me getting chemo, he would be relieved to see me joking around in the treatment room with Lisa and Matt. Jonathan and I usually got along growing up; my first memory is rolling backwards after

he pushed me, and my second is tearing down a poster hanging from his bedroom door. He once pushed me down on my butt so hard that it bruised my sacrum, making me think I broke it. "I have two ass cracks," I said. But we actually had very few fights; confining our competitiveness to trying to get the attention of our young cousins at family reunions and video games.

If I beat him at a video game, he'd throw his controller and storm out of the room.

He was a lot better at being nice to me. We played sports together, with him coaching me to be a better player. He used to be my catcher in the backyard as I practiced pitching for my Little League team. One time the ball I threw bounced off the ground and jacked him in the balls. He used a cup after that.

Once treatment ended, Jonathan and I stopped talking about my cancer altogether and rarely acknowledged I ever had it. I used to think our relationship would be better this way, but now I'm not sure. Is it normal for two brothers to pretend it never happened?

At sixteen, I still wasn't aware of the benefits of having cancer. As we battle nasty diseases, maybe we're not meant to think about what a plus the disease is in expanding our horizons and helping us enjoy the time we have. I believed that thinking that cancer totally sucked was a defense mechanism to help me survive. I didn't fear death. For me, cancer simplified my life by reducing my choices and activities. Cancer deprived me of some things, which then made milkshakes and *SportsCenter* more rewarding.

Going to the movie theater or out to dinner became an event. Before cancer, it was just something you do, but after cancer, it was something truly special. I can still recall each meal: Olive Garden with my mom after Cycle Three; Uno's with my mom and Aunt Florence after Cycle Four, to name two.

After Cycle Five, I went to see *Cast Away* with Jonathan and my

family. I can remember everything about the events that took place. It was Christmas. I wore my white Eddie Bauer sweater and olive green cargo pants. I got up to pee halfway through the movie and wondered if everyone knew I had cancer from one look in a dark theater.

I was so happy that day. I was happy that I finished Cycle Five. I was happy that I was healthy enough to see that great movie with my family. I was happy that my brother was there with us. I was happy with life. You heard correctly—I had cancer, yet was genuinely happy with my life. I was so happy that I almost wanted time to stop. It is times like that I miss so badly now that it hurts.

A week after we saw *Cast Away* was Day Ten of Cycle Five. It fell on my seventeenth birthday. I was neutropenic, and on Day Ten of my other two short cycles, I had been admitted into the hospital, but not on this time. My body temperature stayed normal. I didn't have to go to the hospital. What more could I ask? I enjoyed pizza, gifts and the NFL Playoffs at home.

The Redskins' owner had fired the head coach, Norv Turner, after their 9-7 loss to the Giants four weeks earlier. I was disappointed, since the Redskins were 7-6 and still in playoff contention. They ended up losing two of their final three games and missing the playoffs. That led me rooting for whichever team played the Philadelphia Eagles, one of the Redskins' hated rivals.

On New Year's Eve—the day after my birthday—I had some minor mouth sores, but otherwise I was feeling fine. At halftime of the Philadelphia/Tampa Bay game, the thermometer read 100.1 degrees, nearly as hot as the Eagles defense. Although that's not technically a fever, my parents were concerned. It was almost 6:00 p.m., and my temperature was likely to rise by the end of the night. "Why don't you and Dad head to NIH now?" my mom said.

"Are you crazy? "

"No, I'm not crazy. I was just suggesting they could check you out."

"Why the hell would they do that? I don't have a fever."

"Your temperature could rise. You don't want to be forced to go all the way out there at midnight, do you?"

"I just got off the phone with NIH," my dad said as he entered the kitchen. "The doctor on call thinks it's a good idea for us to come in. He's going to listen to your lungs and get a blood and urine sample. He said that if you seem okay then he'll send us home, as long as you don't get a fever."

"Dammit! It's New Year's Eve, this isn't supposed to happen. I'm at Day Eleven—I thought I was past this part."

"I'll put the game on the radio. Do you want me to fill up a bottle full of Kool-Aid before we leave? It might keep your fever down."

"Yeah."

Jonathan was leaving for a friend's house for the night. "You get back home quickly, and I'll see you tomorrow," he said. "Make sure you drink up your Kool-Aid."

"I'm going to drink the shit out of this."

The game was still in the fourth quarter when we arrived at NIH, the Eagles up 14-3. I had finished the Kool-Aid and gave the nurse the clearest urine sample ever. She drew my blood and sent me to a room of my own. I refused to lie on the bed. I sat in a chair and swung the small TV around so I could watch the end of the game. My dad pulled up a seat next to me when a young doctor came in for my examination. "You sound great," he said. "We'll just wait for your blood results and go from there."

The nurse entered with the results: my ANC was 240, which meant that my counts were rising. She was inclined to let us leave until my dad said, "Benjy, why don't you have her check your temperature one more time?"

I agreed hesitantly, regretted immediately, too shy to take it back. "Hmm, it came up with 100.4." She tried again...same thing.

"I can still go, right?"

"I don't know, let me tell the doctor."

I wanted so badly to leave, yet I knew what the doctor was going to say. "We're going to have to keep you overnight."

"But why? My white cells are already increasing and my fever isn't getting any higher. It's taken the entire day just to reach 100.4."

"I'm sorry, Ben, but you don't want to wake up in the middle of the night really sick, do you? We may get you out of here tomorrow. I'll see you in the morning." The doctor left.

The way I saw those last two days of the twentieth century, I was supposed to get a fever on December 30, on Day Ten with my neutrophils somewhere near zero, as I had in previous cycles. But since Day Ten was my birthday, I was gifted a cool body temperature. That was some kind of destiny.

Then my parents taking me to the hospital on Day Eleven, the nurse taking my temperature, the doctor insisting that I stay, these wrong moves altered the Super Man karma. They were irreparable errors with the result of making me feel less like a Super Man. It messed up my plan for myself.

I was so sad I almost cried, which made me feel worse realizing how much of a pussy I was. My dad tried to lighten my mood. "This is no big deal. You stay tonight and you'll be out of here tomorrow."

"Yeah."

"You'll be alright. I know you're fine, but you know how these doctors are. We'll watch the ball drop later." Missing the New Year's Eve celebration in Times Square was the least of my worries at this point.

"Yeah."

He went to the bathroom, and then Alexis rolled by my room in a wheelchair pushed by her mom, who was wearing a particulate mask. "Hey Ben, how are you?" her mom asked.

"I'm fine, just watching the playoff game. My temperature is 100.4 so

they won't let me leave."

"I'm sorry. I bet you're wondering why I'm wearing this mask. I have a cold and don't want to get Alexis sick."

"Is she neutropenic? She looks sleepy."

"Yes, her counts are low and she isn't feeling well. Alexis was supposed to go to her friend's New Year's party tonight, so she's a little upset. Did you have any plans?"

"No. I knew I'd be neutropenic, so I didn't make any plans," I said.

I could have followed Alexis to her room, but I didn't. I was so sore about not being able to watch Dick Clark's *New Year's Rockin' Eve* at home on my fifty-three inch sweetheart that I didn't try to make my miserable situation better. In my fucked-up rationale there was no point in hanging out with Alexis. Since I couldn't have my first choice—being at home with my flatscreen—I would go with my last choice, which was being in the hospital without any company but my dad. Just as I had starved myself in Cycle Three, this time I subjected myself to the most punishing option–having no New Year's Eve celebration at all.

My temperature went down by itself, just like I knew it would. I turned down the volume on the TV as the Eagles beat the Buccaneers 21-3, got on the bed and fell asleep. It was almost 12:30 when I woke up. "I missed the ball drop? Why didn't you wake me up?" I asked my dad.

"I fell asleep, too."

I turned off the TV and went to sleep without even brushing my teeth. I woke up on New Year's Day energized. I wanted to lie on my couch at home and watch bowl games all day on my huge TV. When the young doctor made his rounds, I was already tying my shoes to go home. "Hey Ben, how are you feeling?"

"Fine. I'm ready to leave."

"Well, your neutrophil count is just over 400. Sorry, but we can't let you go until it reaches 500."

"My blood was taken hours ago. I'm sure my ANC is 500 by now.

How about you check my blood again in an hour, then I can leave."

"No, I don't think so. It's best that you stay here one more day. Let us know if you need anything."

That young doctor became my most hated person alive. I wanted to kill him. My sadness was replaced by so much rage that I was tempted to unhinge my tiny TV and bash his skull in with it. How could he do this to me? He knew I was fine, and he knew my ANC would easily reach 500 later that day. My dad and I watched football. Without ESPN, our game selection was limited, but we did get to see Virginia Tech pound Clemson 41–20 in the Gator Bowl.

The next morning I decided that I was leaving whether or not the doctor authorized it. My neutrophil count was over 2,000 and he had no choice but to discharge me. When I finally got back home, Worm came over to my house to play *Madden NFL 2001* on PS2. He used to have an eight-game winning streak, but since I started playing with the Packers, I had won three in a row. "Terry asked about your surgery," Worm said.

"That was nice. How did she know I was having surgery?"

"I told her."

"What did you say?"

"Well, she was asking about you, and I said, 'Ben is having surgery on his hip to remove the tumor.'"

"What did she say?"

"She said, 'Oh, that's good.'"

I laughed and said, "That's good? I think it might suck."

"She just meant it was good that they were removing it."

I had told only my closest friends when my surgery was scheduled. My No Complaining rule prohibited me from talking about it to people I didn't see all the time—like all females, including Terry. They would only know if somebody close to me told them. They weren't going to hear it from me. Worm beat me and ended my three-game winning streak.

When I returned to school, the halls were gloomy. Things were mov-

ing in slow motion. I tried to listen to people as they talked to me but all
I heard was white noise. I was physically present in my classes, but mentally I was absent. I could only think about tomorrow. Was my surgery
really less than twenty-four hours away?

At lunchtime, I sat in my usual spot next to my friend Nick and
across from Terry and Lily. Lily had a skin tone you can achieve only as a
lifeguard. She gave me the time of day no other girl did, except for those
like Andrea who liked me only for my hair.

I wrote Lily's name in the steam on the shower door, always above
other names that came and went. Hers remained because I wanted her. I
dreamt about being electrocuted in front of her in the school stairwell as
my cancer was destroyed and I transformed into a taller, tanner, curlier-
haired version of myself. I would wish for a time when I could talk to
her as easily as I talked to Nick, or as other guys like Drew talked to her.
I would think for hours of things to say, and then when I saw her and
she smiled and said "Hi Ben!" in her cheery voice, I would be speechless.
I longed for Lily in my pathetically girl-absent life.

Before my visit to the sperm bank, Lily had tried to relax me by saying, I'll carry your unborn child," which then became on ongoing joke.
How about we try one more time for old time's sake?

"Hi Ben," Lily said.

"Hey guys," Terry said upon arrival.

"Hey," I said.

That was all the two girls said to me the rest of lunch. Nick asked
me millions of questions about my surgery and my awesome fifty-three
inch flatscreen. When lunch was over Nick said, "Good luck, Ben. I'll
pray that everything goes well."

Terry and Lily said nothing. No "goodbye" and no "good luck." I
wondered, "How can you sit there and say nothing to me? Do you understand that I'll never be the same after today?"

Of course I knew my cancer intimidated other people. I understood

where their fear came from, but at that moment, I wished someone had the guts to say something. As the years went by, people found other things to talk to me about, but that day, at that table in the cafeteria, everyone knew what was next for me, and not one of the girls said a word.

At the end of the school day, however, when the bell rang after final period, many of my friends wished me luck. Drew bear-hugged me. "I love you, buddy" he said. "Get your ass back to school soon."

My surgery was going to be so early that we decided to stay at Aunt Florence's overnight. At six in the evening, we left for Washington, D.C. Goodbye, House. I had to leave my sweetheart flatscreen behind.

Jonathan was there for me. A couple of weeks earlier, he told me that he wouldn't hesitate to withdraw from Virginia Tech for a semester so that he could be with me. "I don't mind," he said. "I can easily make up one semester."

"I'll be fine. The first few weeks will be difficult, but then things will go back to normal."

When we got to Aunt Florence's house, Jonathan and I watched *Erin Brockovich*, which sucked, and I fell asleep halfway through it half-dreaming:

"What will it feel like to see your little brother all fucked-up tomorrow?" I dreamed I asked.

"What will it feel like to be all fucked-up?" he fired back.

"I don't know. At least I'll be asleep. I won't even know what I look like, but you'll have the image forever. For months, every time you talk to me or look at me you'll be reminded."

"Maybe, so long as you pull through."

"I love you, big brother. You know that, right?"

"Yeah. I love you, too."

It only happened in my head but that's what we could have said, or should have said.

The nurse threaded the IV and gave me a mild sedative. She un-locked the brakes on the bed and guided me down several hallways. My heart pounded so loudly I thought it might explode through my chest. My life would soon be in the hands of other people for several hours. Some serious surgery was about to transpire: cutting, sawing, stitching, stapling, and bleeding. I didn't want to lose the use of my leg, and even more importantly, I didn't want to lose my life.

The nurse eased the bed through the double doors into a large room. I looked to my right and saw Dr. Wodajo preparing instruments. There was a bed surrounded by tables with silvery tools displayed on them. Ev-erything was there except a chainsaw. "Why don't you slide over to the other bed and dangle your feet over the side?" the nurse suggested.

"Okay. What are you doing?"

"I'm going to put in the epidural now."

"Is it going to hurt?"

"Just a pinch."

"Don't worry, Benjamin," my mom said. "I'm here."

"Are you ready?"

"Yeah…that wasn't so bad."

"Hold still so I can secure it…there we go."

"Am I going to need an enema?" I asked.

"No," the nurse replied.

"Good."

"Benjamin, I have to go now," my mom said quietly. "Don't worry, you'll be okay. I love you."

"I love you, too."

"He'll be just fine."

The anesthesiologist said, "What I want you to do is slide your feet onto the bed, and push back a little bit…good. Now, lie down on your back. Don't worry about the needle, that's not going anywhere."

"How's that?" I asked.

"Good."

"Can you tell me before you start the anesthesia so I know when I'm going to sleep?"

"Of course. Now, just relax."

I looked up at the ceiling with three nurses and the anesthesiologist staring down at me. It was like something out of a movie. Then boom, somebody turned off the lights.

I woke up in the recovery room a mess: my left leg was in traction with a large bandage around my hip, my eyes were covered with ointment, a small suction tube was inserted through my nose that went down the back of my throat and into my stomach, an epidural was in my back, three epineurals were feeding pain medication through my hip and into my nerves, oxygen tubes were in both my nostrils, a catheter was coming out of my penis, two IVs were stuck into my right arm, two more IVs into my left arm, and a large breathing tube was shoved down my throat.

I have almost no recollection of what happened next. In my barely-conscious state I noticed the breathing tube, at which point I freaked and began to choke on it. I couldn't say or move anything except my finger, so I tapped my mom's hand. She called over the anesthesiologist. "I think he wants the breathing tube out."

"I can't take it out yet, he just woke up. I'll take it out in a short while."

"Are you sure, because I think he really wants it out."

"I can only remove the tube if he holds his head up for ten seconds."

I heard him loud and clear. I lifted my head away from the pillow and held it suspended as tears streamed down my face.

"Okay, I'll remove the tube," the anesthesiologist said.

I can still remember random events from that day, even though I could barely see and had no concept of time. The first words I spoke were, "Hey Brian Mitchell," when Dr. Wodajo checked on me. In the recovery room my first vomit began immediately after I ate ice chips. I will always

remember the screaming around me: the dude next to me was whining about his leg pain, the girl to my other side screaming as she came out of brain surgery. No amount of opiates in the world could stop her pain.

Dr. Merlin told us the surgery had gone well. He asked me to move my foot from side to side and wiggle my toes. "Oh, I'm so glad to see him do that," my mom said.

"Me too!" Dr. Merlin said.

I asked my mom how many blood transfusions I had received. "We had thirteen people donate for you. You got all of that blood, and still needed one more. Since Jonathan hadn't donated, we sent him down. He was the fourteenth donor."

The volume of blood in fourteen transfusions is more than my body holds, meaning I lost all my pre-surgery blood plus some. I just hoped my dad's blood would not infect me with his love of salmon.

"You had thirteen people give direct donations? Good guess."

Jonathan appeared before me. "Enjoy my blood. It's good stuff," he said.

Jonathan had to return to school for the spring semester. Before leaving he said, "I can still stay if you have changed your mind. I have no problem watching movies with you all day."

"No thanks. The hard part is over with. Plus I get a long break before the next cycle begins."

"Okay. I'll come back home the first weekend you get out of here."

Despite what I told him, I wanted Jonathan to come home with me. At the time I thought I needed him there. If I was this helpless in a hospital, I didn't know how I would manage being at home without him. Would Mom and Dad be able to take care of me by themselves? Would I be able to handle the loneliness? I wasn't about to slow him down by asking him to give up his life for mine. But I had seen how cancer stalled the lives of some of the other guys on the floor, like Charlie and Matt. They were away from home for so long getting treatment that I wondered if their old lives would still be there if they could survive and

get back to them.

A year after my surgery, I asked Dr. Wodajo to send me digital pictures of the operation, and reluctantly, I looked at them. I was split open and the skin was folded down on itself. There were pools of blood and multiple tubes coming in and out. I could see the bone and it was colored blue, the shade of the cancer cells. I was unrecognizable, even to myself.

Each day I recall having had a new visitor, including Mr. Foley, my homeroom teacher, and one of many people who donated blood and platelets. Mr. Foley brought cards that he made all his students write for me, even the ones I didn't know.

Since the age of eight, I have saved every card that was given to me. Even though you would think cards are impersonal, they are not. Aunt Florence always apologized for sending late birthday cards. My parents always wrote, "You are a great son and we love you very much." My brother always finished with his signature logo, "Jonathan Products" written inside a baseball diamond. And Drew's handwriting was always terrible.

I stuck the cards I got after the cancer in my desk drawer with the birthday cards and the Hanukah cards. I stacked them in two piles: cancer cards and everything else. The piles were nearly equal in height, even though one included fifteen years' worth of cards for graduations, holidays and my Bar Mitzvah. Many of them were words of encouragement before my surgery or a show of admiration afterward. The worst ones were blatant praying and pleading that I make it through the cancer experience successfully.

When I was sixteen, I loathed the get-well cards. I didn't need or want that shit—the pity, support, whatever it is that compels people to send cards. I often didn't even read them and just stuck them in my drawer. My mom always said, "I bumped into so and so, and she told me that she's thinking of you and prays for you all the time."

My mom couldn't understand that I didn't need/want/enjoy hear-

ing things like that, and I would cut her off by saying, "I don't care, stop telling me that crap. Did she tell you she's praying for Jonathan? I see no reason why she'd pray for me but not him." Nobody meant to anger me—they just didn't know what else to do. I guess if they had known I was a Super Man, then they wouldn't have thought the prayers and cards were necessary.

Years after my surgery, I read through them. Maybe I was getting soft in my old age of twenty-three, but when I sorted through the cards, they suddenly meant something to me. All those people cared enough to send their thoughts and wishes, and some sent cards monthly, like Drew's parents, or my home school math teacher. My mom's friend, who volunteered at the White House, sent a card signed by President Clinton (a replica, of course.) Drew had passed a card around school when I was first diagnosed and all the kids signed it. My older relatives sent what few thoughts they could muster. My young cousins even contributed some of their artwork.

My parents' friends sent me cards easily. They had been doing it for everyone they knew all their lives. It was sort of a habit with them. Admiration from my friends was more meaningful to me. I recalled how much I wanted Lily and Terry to tell me that they were thinking of me when we had lunch together in the cafeteria the day before my surgery. They were too shy to say it. Cards said what my friends couldn't bring themselves to speak outright. They even gave me cards when they visited the hospital. Sometimes writing is easier than talking.

Worm wrote, "The way you have handled yourself throughout all of this is remarkable. I admire it." I had no idea how my friends felt about me having cancer. Even though he never knew about my Super bone marrow, he still recognized that I was a Super Man. Jonathan left a similar note at the house which I read when I got home. I nearly cried.

Over time I came to appreciate the cards and prayers more, and the

gifts less. At first, I loved the hoards of gifts, everything from magazines to video games. But finally I told my parents, "Tell people to stop sending me gifts, this is getting ridiculous." With my sweetheart fifty-three-inch flatscreen and my PS2 I had all I needed.

Before I left the hospital for home, my nurse pulled out my penile catheter. As my dad had left the room, the expression on his face, said, "Damn, I'm glad nobody is pulling a tube out of my dick. Good luck with that, son."

Then I tried to pee, but nothing came out. The nurse explained that she was reducing my IV hydration rate so that I would have more time before my bladder filled, but when I tried to go for the second time I was still unsuccessful. "Why can't I pee?" I asked her.

"You might have to stand," she said. "When you get physical therapy, you can try again." So when the physical therapist arrived, I asked everyone else to leave the room.

I wanted to try to pee standing up, but since I needed to hold the walker with both hands, I had to have somebody else catch my flow. The nurse accepted my request to hold the urinal directly under my penis. "Like this?" she asked.

"That's fine…dammit, I can't pee."

At this point, I couldn't tell if my inability to urinate is due to a bladder muscle problem or nervousness. After all, this pretty nurse is staring at my junk while her hand is one inch away from my penis. I was surprised I didn't get excited. But, I did not lose my focus because if I couldn't figure out a way to pee, they would insert another catheter, which I did not want.

Meanwhile, to show the physical therapist I could do it, I inched down the hallway. In the background I can hear President Bush being sworn into office on my television. I was just glad my room had ESPN so I did not have to listen to the news. My physical therapist wanted me to switch to crutches, so I tried but took a wrong step and had to place

my left foot down for balance. This frightened me, so I switched back to my walker. I would have liked to impress the PT with my awesome progress, but I was more comfortable on the walker, so when she left, I was right back where I had started when she arrived.

My nurse came in, and I still had not managed to pee. "The doctors are concerned that you have not defecated in ten days," she said. "So I will be inserting a suppository to correct that." She grabbed my left buttock and tilted me so she could push a soft capsule up my rectum. "It can take up to six hours," she said. I might have enjoyed this ass-grabbing under different circumstances, more specifically, without anal penetration.

For the next few hours, I lay waiting for the laxative to work. By then I had to urinate badly. "If you are not able to urinate soon, I can insert a catheter up your urethra."

"While I'm awake? No way," I said, but when I tried to pee again, no success. But four hours have passed since she inserted the suppository and I thought I might be ready to poop. Seconds later, I knew I needed to poop. I had no time to waste. I pressed the call button and two nurses came quickly. "How are we going to do this?" I asked. "Is it going to be possible to poop under these circumstances?" One nurse wrapped her arms around my backside and lifted slightly, just enough for the other to slide the bedpan under my ass.

"I think I may be able to pee," I said.

The nurse with the bedpan grabbed the urinal next to her and maneuvered it under my dick. I let loose. A massive pile of feces exited my body, as well as a dreadful odor. This is the first time in my life I pooped in front of strangers, let alone two girls. I don't even like to take a dump in public restrooms.

When I was done defecating, the nurse to my right continued to hold me above the bed as the other nurse wiped my ass. They lowered me back to the bed. "Nice job!" the first nurse said cheerfully, but I was disappointed that I still couldn't pee.

"Your cousin is here, she's outside the room," the second nurse announced. My beautiful cousin Elizabeth was assigned to watch over me that evening, while my parents went out to celebrate Mom's fiftieth birthday.

"Can you do something about the smell?" I asked my nurse. She found a small spray bottle of Medi-aire: Biological Odor Eliminator. She emptied half the bottle before Elizabeth arrived.

"I have to pee so badly that I want the catheter," I told her as I writhed in agony.

Elizabeth was still waiting outside when an older nurse arrived with a box of catheter equipment: collection bag, rubber tube and lubricant. Without even saying hello, she got down to business. "Take off that sheet and pull your gown to the side."

The pain was excruciating. I had heard that the catheterizing process was easier if you had an erection, but how could anybody could get it up in this situation? When she pushed the catheter through my urethral sphincter, yellow fluid shot through the tube and into the bag. Five minutes later, done peeing, I look up to see my parents had not gone out to celebrate Mom's birthday after all. They had been too worried about me to leave the hospital.

I asked my dad to put on *Ferris Bueller's Day Off* into the VCR. The four of us watched the movie in silence, until Ferris finished his day off. Then I pressed the morphine clicker to help me fall asleep.

Click. Click. Goodnight.

Just like Dr. Merlin said, I was allowed to leave the hospital two weeks later. I didn't feel ready to leave even though I looked forward to wearing normal clothing, especially my favorite yellow Adidas pants.

I rode home in an ambulance. Can we sound the siren just once? Pretty please? The basement would be my residence for the next few months. My dad had already pushed aside one of the couches, and in its place was a hospital bed much like the one at Washington Hospital Center. The bed

was in view of my fifty-three inch sweetheart. The bathroom was down the hall, far enough for me to get some practice on my shiny walker.

My walker would not fit through the bathroom entrance, so my dad removed the door from the hinges, creating a wide-open view of the toilet from the hallway. Every time I heard somebody approaching I yelled, "Keep your eyes straight ahead! No communication, just keep your eyes straight ahead!"

Just as before, I still hadn't realized the seriousness of my surgery. I thought I would quickly get back to the way I was before that grueling tennis match with Friedman nearly a year earlier. You may wonder how I could possibly see it that way, considering one of my body's largest bones had been removed and replaced with nothing. I was a Super Man. That was enough.

When I got home after surgery, I had three weeks before the start of Cycle Six. I was busier than you'd expect. I had daily visits from any combination of a nurse, physical/occupation therapists, and home school teachers. The rest of my days consisted of video games, friendly visits, TV and movies. I lived strictly in my basement where the TV was almost always on and I was usually in the La-Z-Boy my parents got me the previous summer for my confirmation. My life was serene, safe under my parents' care, content on my hospital bed and La-Z-Boy. I shook a noisemaker when I needed my parents. Sometimes I shook it just to bug them. They left urinals next to my bed at night. They set up my sponge bath, and emptied my urinals each morning. They put on my brace and tied my shoes for me. They even inserted my games into the PS2.

I was the only one in the neighborhood with PS2. One afternoon I had five friends at my house playing on four controllers. I was getting at-home physical therapy while they played but I told them when I was done with PT, someone was giving up a controller.

Although I hated the thought of getting more chemo—almost twice

the number of cycles as before my surgery—there actually was a good reason for it. Research showed that the additional cycles would be good insurance against recurrences.

Cycles Six through Eight were all long because the long cycle isn't as hard on the body. Those of us at NIH needed all the healing power possible following our surgeries. I decided to do all three cycles as an outpatient and stay at Aunt Florence's house.

My body didn't like getting more chemo. On the first night back I vomited for what my mom claimed was thirty minutes. My vomits were violent, deafening episodes as I hurled chunks, bile and acid, over and over and over. When there was nothing left to spew, the dry heaves started over and over and over. My body wanted to expel the poison, and if that included part of my intestine as well, then so be it. I sat on the couch hunched over my bucket, as my mom sat next to me ready to switch me for a new container while she emptied the first.

During respites, I looked up at the TV. The University of Virginia basketball team was in the process of beating #3 Duke 91–89, but I contained my joy because Aunt Florence was upstairs intently rooting for Duke because both her kids went there.

After being home for several weeks, I was authorized to shower in place of sponge bathing. My parents bought me a shower chair and a handheld shower head. I wasn't supposed to move without wearing my brace, which kept my leg abducted, so I tried stalling because I didn't know how I would get in and out of the walk-in shower without assistance. But Dr. Merlin had instructed me to thoroughly clean my wound, so I allowed my dad to help me. He insisted that there was no shame in asking for help, even if that meant my own father seeing me naked at seventeen. I recoiled, inexplicably demeaned. For the first time, I felt like an invalid. I was not someone my dad could admire now, and I thought my relationship with my dad would never be the same. I felt our bond was too important to break over a simple shower.

Nonetheless, my parents prevailed because they were scared I would damage my hip. I was, too. To save my face, they arranged a seat and my walker in such a way that I only needed to stand and pivot in order to reach the shower chair. They stood directly outside the doorless bathroom in case I called, but they never once entered.

I safely showered, got back to the seat, and dressed myself. Once clothed, I let them help me into my hospital bed. They placed six blankets on top of me. I couldn't stop shivering.

The next milestone was getting out of the house. Drew, Worm and I went to Hooters for lunch. Some guys from school sat four tables away. Only one congratulated me on a successful surgery. With the addition of my enormous pink and white brace, I looked bionic. The intimidation factor was on full force. I couldn't believe I was wearing this in public. I looked like a bouquet of carnations.

After lunch, we went back to my house. I decided to enter through the front door—even though there were seven steps to the front porch— instead of my usual route through the garage. My dad saw us coming, so he opened the front door and walked outside. "Hey, boys, Benjy, why aren't you going through the garage?"

"I have to learn how to crutch steps someday, right?"

Without realizing that my left foot had not yet cleared the final step, I took my first tumble. My dad caught me before I hit the ground and helped me up. I felt foolish for making a mistake. I wished my dad hadn't seen me fall. He must have felt frustrated knowing how drastic one single slip-up could be to my healing hip, so he yelled at Drew and Worm as if they were to blame. "Don't worry about it. That was my fault," I explained to them once we got inside. "My dad's just scared that I hurt myself."

"Yeah, we know," Drew said.

After that, I got out of the house as often as possible. That very night we went over to Nick's to watch *The Patriot*, and a week later Nick and I went to CVS to flip through the new *Sports Illustrated* swimsuit issue.

Two friends came over every single day to play PS2, and Bently joined us once the wrestling season was over. Because he had broken his thumb, Bently had trouble moving the analog stick on the controller. I have never laughed so hard at another's expense, watching his player move like he had Tourette's.

My parents loved that my friends came over. "You're lucky to have such good friends," they told me as they brought in boxes of Ho Hos and Twinkies for us to demolish. At dinnertime, my parents invited my friends to stay for a meal. The truth is that we had a blast as we played games for hours each afternoon and evening. Each time a new cycle was to start the next day, I would say, "I'm getting chemo tomorrow so you can't come over. I'll give you a call next week." Like it was nothing.

A year later, I talked to Bently about those good old times. "If it hadn't been for you guys, I probably would have lost my mind. I really appreciate you hanging out with me so much."

"Those were some of the best times of my life," Bently said. "When you were off getting your chemo, we didn't know what to do. It was so boring without you."

The only one of my friends who had personal experience with serious illness was Nick. Nick and I have known each other since the fifth grade, but became good friends through long religious discussions during our ninth grade Humanities class. He was Catholic, yet probably knew more about Judaism than I did. Because he had hemophilia, a bleeding disorder, I felt like he understood my trial more than my other friends. He was pretty much the only person I talked to about my disease. Nick had an extensive medical knowledge which I figured he got from his mom, who was a nurse.

Nick picked me up two weeks after finishing Cycle Seven to eat lunch at Taco Bell. "I have something kind of important to tell you," he said on the way.

"I already know…you have a small penis."

"No, it's a little more serious than that."

I thought of the worst-case scenario of what Nick, a hemophiliac, was about to tell me. My heart skipped a beat.

"I have AIDS."

"Bullshit," I snapped back, wishing he were lying.

"No, I'm serious."

"I know you are."

I took a minute to steady myself. "How did that happen?"

"When I was a baby, I was on a hemophilia medicine that was made from blood products. At the time nobody really knew how to screen blood, so my medicine was contaminated with HIV. By the time I was seven years old I had full-blown AIDS."

"Who else knows about this?"

"My family, of course, but you're the first friend I have told. Actually, my parents didn't tell me until I was ten."

"Why didn't they tell you sooner?"

"I wasn't supposed to live very long, so my parents just wanted me to have a happy childhood. When I was still alive at ten, I guess they figured I had a right to know."

"Weren't you taking lots of pills? What did you think they were for?"

"My parents said they were for my hemophilia. I didn't know the difference; I just did what they told me to. They told me to wash my hands before eating, stay away from sick people, take my vitamins, that kind of stuff. They also told me my immune system was weaker than other people's so I had to be careful. They were describing AIDS without naming it."

"How did you take it when they finally told you?"

"Not well. I started crying. But then I told myself that nothing had changed. And it was true—I was living with HIV for seven years. It just didn't have a name. But, I did feel weird after I found out. I felt like everyone knew I had HIV and they were all looking at me funny. I had

my dad pick me up from school the next day because my stomach hurt. I couldn't handle being around people."

"Wow." I was silent for a moment, thinking. "How'd your family deal with it?"

"It was weird at first, but it's cool now. Nobody babies me."

"That's good. So I'm the first friend you have told, huh? What an honor. I'm glad you told me, but why?"

"I don't know. Sometimes I just feel like talking about it, you know? My dad used to tell me to keep it to myself, that nobody else had a right to know. There was also a lot of discrimination back when I was first infected. But recently my dad's been feeling differently. He even encouraged me to tell you."

"I feel bad that I'm the only one who knows. Our friends give me props for taking on cancer, but you have been living with hemophilia your whole life. If you don't tell people what's going on, you won't get the respect you deserve."

"It doesn't matter to me. You deserve all the props; I respect the shit out of what you're going through."

"Thanks, pal. So, do you get pissed at God for allowing this to happen?"

"No. The way I see it is God gave me this disease because he knew that I could handle it. When I found out about your cancer, I felt terrible, but at the same time I was glad it was you because I knew how strong you are. Out of all my friends I knew you'd handle it better than anyone."

"I just see it as bad luck. What about some of the girls at school who cry over the most pointless shit? Would God ever give them cancer or AIDS?"

"Probably not, since they have trouble handling even broken nails."

"How do you keep your family from pitying you?"

"They don't pity me. They respect what I'm going through. My mom's a nurse, remember? You and I are the same—we don't need any pity."

Nick and I jabbered about our diseases through lunch and on the

ride home. It was surprisingly natural, considering I would normally only talk that long about the Redskins' horrendous kicking game or LaVar Arrington's hitting power. I taught Nick about cancer and neutropenia while he taught me about AIDS and viral loads. So long as he had a low CD4 count (a type of white blood cell), it would be possible for him to contract any of twenty-six rare diseases that people with normal immune systems will never know about. Some of these are cancers.

When I asked Nick which of our diseases he would rather have, he said, "People generally will take what they have because they're scared of everything else. But knowing how much AIDS sucks, I think I would rather have your cancer."

I agreed with him. Cancer can be killed. AIDS is a lifelong disease with no cure. As nasty as chemo is, I bet Nick would give anything to have a cure for AIDS, even one as virulent as chemotherapy. The fact that he's lived as long as he has is a miracle. When he was three years old, the likelihood that he'd be alive at seventeen was probably close to zero. Maybe Nick had super powers he hadn't told me about.

After that, Nick and I had many conversations about life that lasted until the sun came up. I guess telling me was okay because since then Nick told a few more of his friends, including Worm and Terry. Maybe seeing how accepting others were of my cancer inspired him to share the enormous burden of carrying around a life-threatening disease. I felt like a piece of shit for accepting the admiration of my friends while Nick had been able to suffer silently for years. Was I weak for receiving credit, even though I didn't want it? As I mulled over Nick's suffering and wondered whether he was more powerful than I was, I didn't sleep well for the next two weeks.

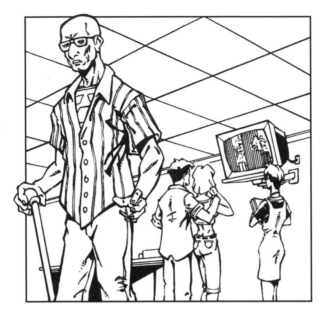

Chapter 5
THE BIG MICROWAVE

A few days later, Dr. Merlin told me I could stop using the brace. I had been doing rehab at Washington Hospital Center the weeks after my surgery. We focused on getting up and down from a chair. Stuff you would think anyone would know were actually complex procedures. Gradually, the therapist showed me how to use the walker for longer distances. I spent hours practicing the correct way to stand at the sink or put on clothes. I was willing to do anything to get stronger.

When I went home, a physical therapist came to my house three times a week. It took many sessions before I could trigger a twitch in my muscles. It was a triumph to slide my leg from side to side on a friction-less surface, or to lift my leg above the bed a fraction of an inch. Though it was painful, I saw results.

At my ten-week post-surgical checkup, Dr. Merlin said, "I want you to start bearing weight on your leg. It'll hurt at first, so start with just putting thirty pounds down."

"If I accidentally step with more than thirty pounds, will it damage anything?" I said.

"No, it's just going to hurt."

"What happens if I fall? Will that do any damage?"

"No, you can fall right now if you want proof."

When I got home, I ripped off the brace and tossed it into the closet. I collapsed on my La-Z-Boy and stretched back feeling total freedom. It took some time to get over the fear of stepping with my left leg. Sometimes I would forget to limit the weight I put on it, and just like the surgeon said, it hurt like hell.

Soon after finishing Cycle Eight in early April, I started intense rehabilitation at my local hospital. My new therapist, Kevin Linde, was short and Jewish like me, so we immediately hit it off. We could always talk about sports, video games and fast cars.

Kevin was from Johannesburg, South Africa. When he was younger he had played many sports—tennis, cycling, gymnastics, and karate—all competitively. He told me about his time in the army, being an electrician and living in Canada where temperatures forty below zero were common.

When you have cancer, people will sometimes tell you things they normally wouldn't. "I was a pyromaniac when I was a kid," he once said. "We had a big field behind our house and in the winter it got very dry. I would set it alight so that I could watch the fire trucks come and put it out. One time I was playing in the back of the house and left something smoldering in the rubber trashcan, and it started burning. Somehow we noticed the huge flame and managed to contain the fire. It could have been really disastrous."

I took oxycodone before our sessions so that I could push through the pain. I made tremendous progress with Kevin's help, and would have

improved even faster if it had not been for the chemo cycles and neutropenia. "Every time I move forward I have to take a chemo break," I complained.

"I guess I'll just have to push you harder when you get back," Kevin said.

The other rehab patients were much older than me and watched curiously as we went through all my exercises, especially re-learning to walk. I walked on an underwater treadmill called an Aqua-Ciser.

Exercising at the local fitness center was more nerve-wracking than rehab at the hospital where everyone had something wrong with him. At the local swimming pool, little kids stared at my scar or gazed at my port. "Keep staring and I'll beat you with my wooden crutch," I would think to myself as I marched past them. It was a great relief to get rid of the port a few months later, but the scar was there to stay. I never said anything to the little kids about it but when I went to the beach the next summer and kids my age were staring, I made up stories to mess with them. "A shark bit me while I was surfing in South Florida. He got me right in the hip, and chewed out the bone. They had to stitch me back together after that. I never went surfing again." Once, some really drunk guys believed the whole story, and kept asking me for more details.

Another story I told about the scar was: "I was at this party with my friend, when he got into a fight. He was getting pummeled until I stepped in. I started punching this guy, when out of nowhere, this big dude slashed me with a knife. He sliced right across my side, from front to back. I had blood pouring out of me, but I still managed to kick his ass. Then, a third dude approached me with a gun and shot me right in the chest near my shoulder. They took me to the hospital, after that." You would have had to be on mushrooms to believe that story, but I loved to tell it.

Because I had to limit the weight on my left leg, I was walking on the handrail platform at the hospital. Whenever I took a step with my left leg, I would hold the rails to remove some of the force. As the weeks

passed, I needed to brace myself less and less. This time, I raised both arms out to the side and took a step…then another. "Look!" I said to make sure I wasn't seeing things.

No crutch, no brace, no handrail, just normal walking. It wasn't quite as good as the Redskins winning the Super Bowl, but slightly better than seeing Jessica Alba in a bikini. "From now on, use one crutch," Kevin said. By the end of June, I ditched my crutch in favor of a cane, and by year's end I was walking with no tool at all.

That spring, Bently and I skipped our last two classes to see *Spider-Man* the day it opened. We spent the whole hour of Mr. Foley's home-room planning precisely when to leave, who would exit first and synchronizing our retreats. Our plans were unnecessary. It turned out security could care less, so weeks later we nonchalantly dipped out to play golf and see *Attack of the Clones*. We left our calculus homework assignments with Nick to turn in for us. I attached a note to our teacher that read: "I had to go see *Spider-Man*. Please don't punish me. Actually, today is my last day of physical therapy. After fifteen-and-a-half months, I'm finally done." I finished the note with a smiley face.

Kevin decided I had nothing more to gain from physical therapy. I told him I would be back when Dr. Merlin cleared me to run again. "You can help me with my running gait," I said. I was still clueless that running was never going to be part of my life again.

Dr. Merlin always had his entourage with him during our visits. As he tested my strength and mobility, he would talk proudly about me to them in Doctor Speak. I knew I was his star patient because he had Dr. Wodajo film me walking and shot pictures of me. Dr. Merlin's confidence was contagious. He thought he was the best surgeon in the world, and the way I deconstructed his bragging to the other docs, he thought I was the best patient ever.

During one checkup, while doing leg extensions, I was trying to show off. I put all my energy into one huge leg lift and I squeaked one

out. I couldn't help it. I got some giggles and one comment: "Too much pressure, huh?"

Another time, Dr. Wodajo said, "Pull your knee up to your body."

"How is that?" I said. "That's about as far as it goes."

"That's great," he laughed. "I can't even do that."

It wasn't as easy for the other patients. Alexis joked that Dr. Merlin was not only unimpressed with her, but that he disliked her. "Dr. Merlin doesn't want to see me anymore," she said.

"Are you serious?" I asked. "I still see him every three months."

"I think he was pissed because I slacked on my ankle stretches."

I told my parents that there should be a poster of me on his walls: Be the best patient you can be. Be like Ben Rubenstein. Dr. Merlin praised me, and for that, I loved him. Seeing him drool over my progress made all the pain I went through, as well as the three-to-four hour nap in the waiting room, worth it. I wanted to be the best and it was hard given how little of my hip was left. Nearly my entire left iliac wing was removed up to the joint, as well as part of my sacrum, and some muscles and tendons. My hip muscles were reattached to others in my abdomen, lower back and butt with dozens of staples and some tape. Why not superglue? My scar is fifteen inches long and it took fifty staples to keep it closed.

Without a bone to stop its migration, my femur—that's the thigh bone—shifted up, causing my left leg to be higher off the ground than my right leg. It gives the perception that my left leg is shorter. To balance things out, even today I wear a two-inch lift in the bottom of my left shoe, though the true discrepancy is over two-and-a-half inches. Obviously they always ask me to remove my shoes at airports because it looks like I could fit a rocket in there.

My body has compensated. Forces normally sent through my hip have been transferred elsewhere. My gait has changed. This bothers me, and to this day, I still try to walk straighter. All these years later, Dr. Wodajo says it's amazing that I can still walk pain-free.

My hip was quirky:

- I felt knee pain referred from my hip anytime my knee was elevated above my hip joint.
- The entire left side of my left leg was completely numb. I now have some feeling.
- I could feel either staples or bone fragments under my skin near my hip flexors.
- When I rubbed the left side of my lower back, I felt it in my penis.
- My left leg would never be nearly as strong as my right.
- When I stood on both legs to pee, the stream stuttered. I usually stand with my left heel slightly raised, like a dog.

I will always have an obvious limp. Bently said, "Turn it into a strut. Then you'll be as cool as a pimp."

My first day back to school after being absent for three and a half months felt strange, like I was an outsider in my native land. Many of my friends welcomed me back, but nobody did it like Bently. At lunch, Bently ran through the cafeteria with a big sign, acting like a cheerleader. The sign had a picture of two ass cheeks labeled "Cancer," and a boot kicking them labeled "Benjy." At the top, it read, "Welcome Back. Way To Kick Cancer's Ass."

My treatment was approaching the finish line, and with only six cycles left, I remember thinking, "I can see the end of the road. I'm almost there." I chose to do the final six cycles as an inpatient. I was tired of schlepping to NIH. Chemo was terrible so I wasn't about to make a vacation out of it. Plus, Barney, Aunt Florence's dog, wanted his couch back.

I became familiar with Bob Barker's irritableness. I relished any time I could watch sports, especially an *NBA on NBC* Tripleheader where I saw Dirk Nowitzki get his tooth knocked out. I noticed the incisor fall to the court live. Then it was shown in super-slow motion, circled in yellow.

I watched dozens of movies in a semi-conscious state, after chemo or Benadryl or who knows what else. I viewed my favorites like *Armageddon* and *Happy Gilmore*, and others I had never seen before like *Copland* and *National Lampoon's Christmas Vacation*. I remember how sad Sylvester Stallone's performance was, and how hilarious Chevy Chase was, but can't describe much more than that. I even got some of my doctors and nurses to watch a few minutes here and there, forgetting, if only temporarily, that their jobs were as serious as my cancer. Those actors and athletes made living with cancer easier than it could have been, and for that I thank them all.

I watched so many games with my dad that I practically memorized commercials. We would see who could name the commercial first, and I always beat him. I was so good that I could win with my eyes closed. After that spring, it just didn't feel right watching sports without my dad next to me. Life went on and on.

By July, my bone marrow had been severely ravaged by twelve cycles of chemo, so I knew Cycle Thirteen, my final short cycle, would be my most arduous yet. Even expecting trouble, I foolishly allowed myself to become constipated. It happened at the worst possible time, when my white blood cells were in free fall. Hard stools can cause a laceration in the rectum, which can open the door to infection. If you have a laceration and you're neutropenic, your rectum won't heal until your white blood cells rise. I had several rectal tears, known as fissures. During physicals I would say, "My butt hurts."

"Let's have a look," Christine would say as she closed the curtain to give me privacy. I would drop my pants, get on the table and lie on my side with my knees in. Then she'd enter and close the curtain behind her. "Let's have a peek." She'd pull down my boxers, spread my cheeks and give my asshole a thorough investigation. "You have an anal fissure at twelve o'clock." Not good.

I was admitted at NIH with a fever. My roommate, Bruce Abraham,

who was in his twenties, had been in the Air Force. "What cycle are you up to?" I asked him.

"I'm at Cycle Three. How about you?"

"I only have one left. How's your treatment been so far?"

"When my port was implanted, my lung got punctured. I had a tube through my chest for three weeks. I was on morphine to stop the pain. The combination of morphine and chemo kept making me puke. I couldn't eat anything and lost twenty pounds."

I just didn't have the energy to be sympathetic to him. Following my penile catheter incident, tubes inserted through any organ made me shiver. I had a nasty anal tear caused by constipation, and all I could do was wait it out. I tried to correct the constipation by taking extra Colace, which gave me diarrhea. I kept pooping, irritating my rectum more. Eventually, I needed oxycodone around-the-clock just to lie in bed.

My platelets dropped to eight thousand. I needed a transfusion. Platelets, like red and white cells, are produced in the bone marrow. They stop bleeding by forming blood clots. When you don't have enough, you may bruise easily, develop nosebleeds or have prolonged bleeding from a cut. This condition can be serious, especially if you bump your head because of the possibility of internal bleeding. Although eight thousand platelets per cubic millimeter of blood may sound like a lot, a normal amount is at least 150 thousand.

Elizabeth and my mom were chatting across from me when I started to feel funny immediately after the transfusion began. "Benjamin, are you alright?" my cousin asked.

"I don't know. I got hot all of a sudden. And I can hear my heartbeat in my head. It's really loud."

My nurse stopped the platelets and switched me to saline. My strange sensations went away a few minutes later, but it would take consolation from Dr. Springs and an IV dose of Ativan to calm me down.

"I'm not getting any more transfusions," I said.

"That was just one platelet sample, it won't happen again," Dr. Springs said. "You really need a platelet transfusion."

"How do you know I won't get another reaction?"

"It's unlikely."

It was later discovered the platelets were contaminated with something akin to food poisoning, but it was better than being contaminated with HIV. Sorry, Nick. I agreed to receive a different platelet transfusion later that afternoon without any problems.

My mom was irate. "That was one time I turned into a raving lunatic," she admitted later. My contaminated platelets came from Walter Reed Army Medical Center in Washington, D.C. As her story goes, I had three direct donation platelets at NIH, although at the time the blood bank supervisor claimed there weren't any. Of course, they happened to appear in the blood bank the following day when it was time for my second transfusion. In the words of my former favorite wrestler, The Rock, my mom laid the smack down on his candy ass.

My roommate for Cycle Fourteen was Joe Curtis, an annoying boy about thirteen. He whined. His mom did everything for him. He never stopped puking and the noises he made kept me awake. I annoyed him right back with my spit bucket. During chemo, swallowing made me nauseous, so I constantly spat. My mom urged me to let her empty the container, but I wanted to see if I could fill it to the brim.

Finally, in early August, I watched the last drop of chemo enter my bloodstream. After ten months of allowing the most toxic liquid any human being voluntarily injects into his or her body, I was done. My nurse threw my last empty bag into the biohazard receptacle. That's it, no more chemo ever again.

The doctors and the staff presented me with a banner they signed that read, "Congratulations Ben!" I didn't want them to ever forget that I was the teenage patient who physically and psychologically kicked the shit out of bone cancer to an extent they'd never before seen. In my

mind, ending chemo was going to be a major accomplishment, worthy of a Diddy yacht party, but when it actually happened, it was a big nothing. I had to begin radiotherapy just three days later.

NIH wrote the book on scaring patients and their families. I think that ability to instill fear was a prerequisite to working there. I figured out their tactics fast, but my parents never did catch on. The docs told us that chemo kills skin cells and makes it easier for the sun to cause damage. So, in late March, when I was crutching around our cul-de-sac on a cloudy, cool day Jonathan came out saying, "Benjamin, you might want to go inside. Mom is going crazy."

"What?"

"She keeps screaming that you're not wearing sunscreen and the sun is dangerous."

"It's March, and I have been out outside for five minutes."

"I know, she's crazy. She has just lost it."

Certain health-related situations trigger something in my mom's brain that causes insanity. In this instance, NIH had convinced my mom that I was going to get skin cancer. I knew I had to be careful, but five minutes in March could certainly do little harm. But my mom was the perfect NIH disciple, swallowing their dire warnings whole.

I may not have tanned in the summer of 2001, but I sure got cooked.

In order to leave my hip joint intact, my surgeon, Dr. Merlin, had not been able to remove the bone margins that have been proven most effective to completely excise the tumor. For that reason, I needed radiotherapy. Christine explained the concept of margins to me: "If you dropped a bucket of sand in the same spot, most of the particles would clump together, but some would fall away. Cancer cells aren't much different. Your iliac crest was the cancer nucleus, but there was no way to tell how far some of the individual cells had wandered."

The Radiation Oncology department was in the bowels of the building. From the main elevators, I went down a long corridor with research

rooms on both sides. Halfway down the hallway were two more elevators. I took one down to basement Level Three, the bottom floor. Once
down there, I turned right and walked down a second long corridor. At
the end was Radiation Oncology. The waiting room was past the recep-
tion desk and down two more small hallways. From there, the nurse took
me into the radiation room, which had a huge machine and a table in
the middle. There was only one door to get in and out of the room. It
must have been a foot thick.

Radiotherapy is a scary process—beams of concentrated X-rays
shooting through parts of your body at different angles. Side effects
from radiation can include short or long-term skin damage, diarrhea, a
decrease in bone marrow production, fatigue, hair loss, nausea, vomiting,
and inflammation of the bladder or rectal lining.

To be certain the radiation is delivered in the same place each session,
permanent tattoos are given to the patients. "Lie on the table and pull
your pants down," the technician said. "Are you ready?"

"Yeah, go ahead."

She reared back and jammed what looked like a Bic pen into my skin
six times. My blue dots were nowhere near as fashionable as the Brahma
Bull inked on The Rock's arm. I pondered getting a better tattoo when
the radiation was over. Breast cancer survivors get one like a pink ribbon
or a flower, a symbol of their strength and courage. I could have gotten
a tattoo to show that I am part of the cancer survivors' club. I thought
about it. It would have to be manly, like a flaming, bloody tumor with a
giant Rambo knife sticking out of it. I decided against it later, because
maybe my fifteen inch surgical scar is admired by everyone.

I went to NIH for radiation every weekday for five consecutive weeks,
for a total of twenty-five sessions. It was a lot of driving, especially considering the radiation process lasted only fifteen minutes. The trip each way
took an hour. It was three weeks before I convinced my parents to let me
drive there myself. They were convinced—more NIH scare tactics—that

radiation aimed at my hip would cause mental fatigue.

I love to drive. I was a speed demon from the get-go, driving, on average, twenty miles per hour over the limit. The police call my kind of driving "reckless." I once reached 101 in a fifty-mile-per-hour zone and seventy-two in a twenty-five-mile-per-hour zone. I liked to roar past other cars by going thirty or forty miles per hour faster than they were going. I drove by my theory of constant acceleration: as long as there was open road in front of me, I was going to go faster. I liked the excitement and the adrenaline rush. I liked being the only one of my friends with the balls to do it. And I liked acting illegally.

Jonathan warned me that I could easily get a ticket, but I wasn't going to slow down until I got caught. To my own surprise, I drove like this for five-and-a-half years before getting a speeding ticket. My CopDar, a gut feeling that a cop was around, worked like a charm.

You may be thinking, "What moron would fight for his life against cancer, and then immediately risk his life on the road?" I didn't see cancer as a fight for my life. I saw it as a collection of mutated cells growing in my hip that had to be killed and removed through a complex regimen of drugs, needles, blood transfusions and checkups. Add to that, I didn't see driving fast as risky. My dad had trained me to be a defensive driver. "Stay five miles under the limit, with no radio and no waving," he instructed me. He required me to accumulate a hundred practice hours before I could go for my license. I even represented my high school in the district safe driving competition. Bently, who exceeded me by making it into the state-level competition, was in three auto collisions in high school.

When I arrived for my first radiation session, a nurse escorted me to the big microwave. Once I maneuvered in the right position, I stayed motionless. I did not want those energy waves anywhere near places they didn't need to be. The nurse left the room and closed the mammoth door behind her, leaving me all alone. The machine made noises and I think it moved around. I couldn't see what was happening because I

had buried my face in a pillow. I was supposed to be scared of radiation, but I never was. Marinate me, baby. I learned to take a nap as the beams cooked and mutilated my cells. Sometimes it felt warm, but that was all there was to it.

My radiation oncologist must have spent hours designing my treatment plan. He showed me the diagram he had made. There were beams coming in from multiple angles, covering a large area from the top of my thigh to the bottom of my ribcage. My radiation dose was moderate—4,500 rads—delivered to my hip joint, the remainder of my ilium and sacrum, the top of my femur, and part of my bowel.

Different organs and tissues can tolerate varying amounts of radiation, which is why the radiation was dispersed. Radiation and chemo are amazing in the sense that they kill cancer and other cells that divide quickly. But, they can also create new cancers down the road. I was given a five percent chance of developing a soft tissue tumor fifteen to twenty years later.

With radiation, my skin changed color to a red so bright that it frightened my friends. I had also developed diarrhea, which intensified to the atomic variety. Since it took over an hour to get home, I often pooped before leaving NIH—just in case.

The bathroom was large for one person. After pooping one afternoon, I rested a couple of minutes before cleaning up and going home. That's when a man walked in: I had forgotten to lock the door. He was a large guy, probably in his forties, and somewhere around 5'11" and 240 pounds. He wore a shirt and tie. He opened the door and turned ninety degrees to his left, at which point he had a direct view of me and my junk.

Instead of simply saying "Whoops," and walking out like a normal person, this fellow stuck around. He was silent. The door closed behind him. We stared at each other for multiple seconds. I can't remember exactly what came out of my mouth, but I know it was along the lines of "Dude!" or "Dude?" It might even have been "Dude, get out, I'm taking a shit here!"

TWICE

A week later, my senior year of high school began. I still had seven more radiation sessions left. My parents wanted me to get tutoring until radiation was complete, but I refused. By the end of the first week of classes, I was exhausted, yet still determined to attend school.

One day I arrived at school early and saw Bently in the lobby. "Dude, I only have two more radiation sessions, then I'm cancer-free."

"That's awesome," he said with a high five.

"Cured" is not a term oncologists use lightly. When someone finishes treatment, the cancer is said to be "in remission," meaning it can come back. Within the first five years following treatment, the term "cancer-free" is used. At the five-year mark, cancer survivors can say that they're cured, even though many survivors and doctors are still reluctant, like the word "cured" is the growth factor a tumor needs for its second wind.

I heard the announcement in my second period physics class. "Two planes have crashed into the World Trade Center towers, one at 8:45 and another at 9:03 this morning," our principal told us over the intercom. Twenty minutes later he came on to make a second announcement. A plane had crashed into the Pentagon, down the road from our school. The place went bananas. We all knew people who worked at the Pentagon and many students had parents who worked there. The guidance office was packed.

It was almost impossible to make a phone call. After lunch, I finally reached my mom. "Benjamin, come home after school, NIH is closed," she said.

"What? You mean I can't get radiation this afternoon? I only have two sessions left."

"Nobody's there, they sent all Federal employees home."

"All right. What about tomorrow? Can I get radiation tomorrow?"

"I doubt it."

"Dammit, I just want to get this over with."

Nick came over to my house to watch the news after school. "I can't

believe this shit. I just feel sad right now," he said.

I could not feel the same way as everyone else in the country did. People expressed all kinds of emotions—sadness fear, anger and disgust— but the emotion I felt most was disappointment. I wanted my treatment to be over and I had not gotten my penultimate dose of radiation. Nick and I watched footage of the twin towers crumbling over and over again. I had never seen anything like that, and it was mesmerizing to watch it unfold right in front of my eyes.

I felt hollow, like the title character in one of my favorite shows, *Dexter.* Trauma as a little boy made Dexter into a psychopathic serial killer—"a monster," he calls himself. Dexter kills out of need. Dexter questions whether he can change into the person he was supposed to be had the trauma not occurred. In the end, he can't. A monster is who he is.

My need to hold in my emotions was a factor in the creation of my Super Man complex. I shut down all my feelings to help me get through the early weeks of cancer. But denying any emotional response was like eating cherry Twizzlers: once I started, I couldn't stop. I eliminated fear and sadness from my consciousness. I came as close as any sane guy can get to thinking he can deflect bullets. Imitating Superman boosted my self-esteem. Feeling invincible fed my ego. The more deluded I became about my super powers, the more I was able to cope with the inconveniences of cancer. Like Superman himself, I became detached, the resident of another world.

Unlike Dexter, I never made a conscious decision to be the way I was. I didn't get to consider if I was better off as a Super Man. A Super Man was who I was now. After Nick went home, my mom came downstairs, visibly upset. "Benjamin, I have some terrible news," she said.

"What is it?" I asked hesitantly.

"I just got off the phone with Alexis's mom…Matt passed away four days ago."

"What? That's not possible; he finished treatment months ago and

was doing so well. What happened?"

"He developed an infection in his artificial rib cage and went in for surgery, but then developed a large blood clot. NIH is having a memorial service for him this Sunday."

Now, despite my intention of being invincible, I struggled to hold back tears. I went up to my room so that Mom couldn't see me shaken. Matt was the only cancer patient I had considered a friend. Yet I didn't even know him that well because my Super Man complex would not allow me to open up to other Sick Kids. I keep thinking about Dexter.

Dexter is unable to reach out to people close to him out of fear that he'll hurt them. I couldn't reach out for fear of being seen as the Sick Kid. I needed people to see me as a Super Man. Dexter was empty by nature; I had made myself hollow by a subconscious force. The shrinks call this an attachment disorder. I call it a survival technique. With Matt dead, I had to work overtime to keep my feelings for him from flowing out. I thought about his life.

He had been a mechanic in the Army when the docs diagnosed him with pneumonia, without even taking an X-ray. Then he lost feeling in his shoulder and arm, and now the docs said it was pneumonia plus a bug bite.

When Matt began to vomit blood, the docs finally took an X-ray. What they saw was cancer. They evacuated him to Walter Reed hospital, and then to NIH for special treatment.

When in the treatment room together, Matt and I would joke around and find humor in our own fucked-up cancer stories. We talked about baseball and how he'd have to learn to throw with his left arm since cancer had taken ribs and his lung on his right side.

"When I finish chemo, I'm going back to upstate New York. I'm going to drink beer and go fishing every day. I can't wait." This is what he told me right before he finished treatment, the last time I saw him.

Matt always called his artificial rib cage his "Auto Bondo Body," because the material was similar to the putty used in chassis repair. He

and Charlie didn't take life too seriously. They used to take midnight post-chemo trips to Krispy Kreme, packing the car with anyone willing to join them, and ordered dozens of doughnuts each. They then drove back to NIH and puked Krispy Kremes all night.

They'd compete to have the lowest ANC, and the longest and freaki-est surgery. When Charlie's leg surgery went thirteen-and-a-half hours, Matt begged his surgeon to prolong his for fourteen hours. The surgeon said there was no way he could go over six hours. That's when Matt negotiated with him to keep a piece of his cancerous rib in a jar. He car-ried that rib around with him like a trophy. Matt and Charlie had unique ideas on how to cure cancer, like drink alcohol until the tumors were saturated, or thread electrical wire into them.

One patient on the floor had cancer that caused him to go blind just before getting his driver's permit, a source of immense frustration to him. On Christmas Day, when the NIH parking lot was deserted, Matt and Charlie took this blind patient out for his first drive. The car lunged, jerked, sped, spun doughnuts and occasionally hit snow banks. Blues Brothers music blared out the open windows while Matt and Charlie shouted directions, laughing wildly.

Matt had driven down from upstate New York the day before the surgery to correct the infection in his Auto Bondo Body. He stayed with Charlie. He coughed all night while Charlie pounded his back trying to dismantle the congestion. Just before his operation, Matt told his doc he didn't feel well and closed his eyes. Charlie waited as the doc frantically tried to save him. Then he sat with Matt until he passed. With Matt gone, I think Charlie lost the will to fight. My unwillingness to feel emotion for my friends was not changed by how much I missed Matt.

I saw Charlie at Matt's memorial service and he didn't look well. We talked about PS2, and then I went home. I had a policy of not staying in touch with other cancer patients, so I didn't know that Charlie's cancer had never gone away, even after treatment. That was the last time I saw

Charlie. As with Matt, it was only after his death that I was able to admit how much I liked the guy.

Not even Matt could rival Charlie's goofiness. Charlie once put his finger up his nose during a scan. Then he frantically brought the film to Lisa proclaiming that the scan showed a serious problem. Lisa, who was very fond of him, called the doctors over to take a look. When the doctors checked it out, they missed his prank entirely. Charlie finally explained to them what he had done, and as they caught on, they laughed as hard as he did. It took Lisa a few days to forgive him.

I had met Charlie on my first visit to NIH, virtually mute because I was so overwhelmed. Charlie cajoled me until he managed to get a laugh out of me, and then welcomed me to the group the same way he did for everyone else. He was the life of the room no matter where he was.

Charlie had suffered for months at an Army hospital in South Carolina losing seventy pounds. First he was diagnosed with shin splints and then with compartment syndrome, where compressed nerves damage muscle and impede blood flow. Both diagnoses were totally bogus, so his mother enlisted their Congressman to intervene. Once Charlie was transferred to private care, he was diagnosed with cancer. The private physician was amazed at how big Charlie's tumor was. Because of the treatment delay, his cancer had already invaded his lymphatic system. Charlie was given less than a ten percent chance of surviving six weeks, but he persevered for two years.

Dr. Merlin recommended amputation, but Charlie convinced him to salvage his leg in what must have been an impossible decision. After surgery, he received a radiation dosage that left his flesh crispy-charred black. He began walking again two weeks after his surgery and throughout radiation. I watched Charlie handle all of this with complete composure. He might have had a few super powers himself.

At the end of his life, his mother told me, Charlie slept most of the time while a constant parade of friends and family visited. The night he passed, he sat up and pointed to the door, and said, "Matt's here!" He

then drew his last breath.

"Charlie and Matt are probably up there cracking jokes about us right now," his mother said. Sadly, I was unaffected, while everyone else struggled in the wake of his death. The head of pediatric oncology stormed out of the memorial service in tears. I was worried that Alexis was going to have a hard time without Charlie, just as Charlie had lost a lot of his will to live when Matt died. I wasn't part of that: my identity as a Super Man had prevented me from getting close to other cancer patients, even if they were as cool as Matt and Charlie.

Just like that it was all over. Despite missing my September 11 radiation treatment, I finished and officially became cancer-free on September 14, 2001 at approximately 3:40 p.m.—exactly one year after Phase II of my life began, almost to the minute. I always found that interesting. Not symbolic, just interesting. One minute I was the perfect cancer patient with the superhuman ability to battle a nasty disease, and the next minute I was a Cancer Survivor. This was the moment I had been waiting for, ever since Dr. Springs said to me, "You have Ewing's sarcoma."

My cancer was officially in remission, and life could go back to normal. Normal was what I hoped for and expected. I strove to finish each day without thinking about cancer even once. I thought something dramatic might accompany the freedom from cancer, but nothing really changed. My left iliac wing didn't suddenly grow back, and the months lost at NIH were gone forever. Having cancer was similar to not having cancer—they were both part of the gradual path known as my life. Events occur, milestones are reached, and life just keeps moving along.

Rick Dollack invited me to a party at his house the night I became cancer-free. I had known Rick for years but I had never hung out with him outside of school. When I arrived at his house, everyone was out on his deck listening to Outkast's "Bombs Over Baghdad". When the verse "Cure for cancer, cure for AIDS" played, Worm cranked up the volume.

"That one's for you, Benjy," he said.

Even though I was surprised at what a big nothing becoming a survivor is, my family was hot on the idea. My mom wanted to have a survival party, and bothered me until I agreed to celebrate at Pizza Hut, which I called the, "Cancer Raping Celebration Dinner," or CRCD. My mom made a big deal about it, but I acted modestly. Aunt Elsa sent me a $50 gift certificate to Outback Steakhouse for finishing treatment. I saved it for a special occasion, like taking Jessica Alba on a date. I ended up using it for my first anniversary of surviving cancer because Jessica had never returned my calls. I was glad that my relatives made a fuss because secretly, I wanted CRCD to be a national holiday with a parade down Pennsylvania Avenue where I would stand next to George W. Bush on a float, smiling and waving to the hoards of excited supporters.

Still there was some extra attention. When our journalism teacher, who was pregnant, mentioned having morning sickness, Worm butted in. "Oh yeah? Well, Ben just survived cancer."

"You win," the teacher laughed. Later, the class invented a character for my tumor, named Ewing Sarcoma, which looked like a bearded SpongeBob SquarePants and had a British accent. "Jolly ho, Benjamin. Why don't you bloody like me, anymore? I gave you so much joy in your life; the least you could do is take me back. Fine chap, I'm going to run along with the other tumours now."

Other things had changed besides having the honor of hanging out with Rick. Some friends had begun drinking. Others were dipping, or using spit tobacco. One guy was in rehab in California. I was surprised when my former tennis partner, Friedman, landed himself a girlfriend. It baffled me since we both used to pee ourselves around girls. He had transformed to be one of my most outgoing friends. But I couldn't relate to him now that I didn't play tennis anymore. I was changing too. My eyebrows started growing back. When Drew noticed he asked, "Dude, are your eyebrows blond?"

"Looks like it."

"Is your hair going to come in blond?"

"I don't know. I have heard stories about people's hair growing back differently. Like, some people had straight hair and it grows back curly."

I delayed my senior picture until I had normal eyebrows and eyelashes, both of which returned to my normal brown color. But in the most unfair event yet, my beautiful curly hair didn't come back. I prayed for my hair to return. It was the only time in my life that I felt God, as opposed to simply chanting Hebrew that was written in my prayer book. I had faith God would save me from a lifetime of devastation. He would show his love for me by restoring my locks.

I waited for the thousands of strands to break through my scalp and create curls that Andrea could play with once again. I waited for days, then weeks, then months, then years. Is it possible that chemo sped up what was genetically predetermined? I'm still waiting for "the monster on top of my head," as my uncle described it, to grow back. It can take nine years for hair to grow back after chemo, right? In my defense, and in accordance with the theory that it's more socially acceptable to be hairless resulting from cancer than genetics, much of my hair elsewhere also failed to grow. Without close inspection, it might appear that I shave my legs and armpits.

When I was first diagnosed with cancer, Rick had presented me a gift, a video with a highly complex plotline titled *Hot Pink #19*. Before my surgery, I had let Worm borrow it. After he had returned it, I had noticed that the clear piece of plastic covering the film was missing. One night, I pushed the tape into my TV/VCR, which made a funny noise and then switched off. I turned the TV back on, but it immediately shut off again after another strange sound. "Oops. What the hell do I do now?" I thought.

In Mr. Foley's class the following day, I told my friends of my problem. "*Hot Pink #19* is stuck in the VCR, thanks to Worm."

"I didn't do anything," Worm said.

"Bullshit. You messed up the tape."

"It worked fine for me."

"Nevertheless, I now have a problem. I have to remove that thing or else my parents are going to find it."

For the rest of class, Drew, Worm and I devised a scheme to retrieve the broken video. We called our mission, "Operation: Hot Pink #19," aka, "Operation: Porn Retrieval," aka, "Operation: Ben Is a Perv," aka, "Operation: Masturbation," aka, "Operation: Let's Save Ben's Ass Before his Parents Find Out He has Porn Stuck in his VCR."

That afternoon, Drew and Worm came to my house with a couple of screwdrivers. As I stood lookout, they removed the TV's back panel and attempted to pull the tape out. "How's it going?" I whispered.

"Give us a second," Drew said. "We just started here. Is anyone coming?"

"No, nobody's coming. Wait…nope."

"You asshole. Keep watching."

As the minutes dragged on, I became worried that my dad would walk up the stairs and wonder why Drew and Worm were in my bedroom while I was standing out in the hallway doing nothing. Each time I heard a noise I would say, "Quickly, he's here…no, never mind."

"Ben, how can we work under this kind of pressure?" Worm asked.

"Just do it," I said.

One minute later Drew said, "Well Ben, if the tape wasn't broken before, it definitely is now."

"Did you guys figure it out?" I asked.

"No. It's stuck, so we hit it several times with the screwdrivers."

Just then, I really did hear somebody walking up the stairs. "Hey, my dad's coming," I whispered. I closed my bedroom door and stood in the kitchen pretending to look for food.

"Hey Benjy," my dad said.

"Hey Dad."

"Where are your friends?"

"Oh, we're watching TV in my room, I'm just getting snacks."

My dad ate two pretzels and went back downstairs. I went into my room and said, "That was a close one."

"You are the worst lookout ever!" Worm said.

"Whatever, you guys didn't do too well yourselves."

They had reassembled the TV so as not to draw attention to what they were doing. Because of my dad's routine house checks, I knew that he'd eventually find the tape. Later that night, I used an envelope opener to scrape off the *Hot Pink #19* label and broke the video even more. No way this would play now.

In my opinion, my dad has borderline OCD. He often goes through the house making sure objects are in their proper location. My mom once told me about a most peculiar OCD event. "The other day, Dad realized that I left the visor down in the van," she said. "So he went out and put it back up."

"You mean the next time he drove somewhere, right?" I said.

"No. I mean he immediately walked outside, unlocked the van and put the visor up."

A week after our failed mission, I was watching TV in the basement when my dad shouted, "Hey Benjy, come up here!"

My dad had discovered my broken TV/VCR, just like I knew he eventually would. I joined him in my bedroom and pretended that it was no big deal. "Oh yeah, that's all messed up. I borrowed a video from my friend, but it was kind of broken. He said it would still work, but I guess it screwed up the TV."

"Sure did. I'll have to take this to the shop to get fixed."

During the next week I was antsy, wondering if the TV repairman was able to see the lesbian threesome. Nick worried me even more by saying, "Did you scrape off the label in the front?"

"What do you mean?"

"Some videos have two labels, one on the top and one on the front plastic cover."

"I don't think it had one on the front. What if it did?"

One evening my dad arrived home from work carrying my TV/VCR back into my bedroom. "They fixed it," he said.

"Oh yeah? That's good."

"Let me show you something," he said. Was there a second label?

"You see this tape?" he asked, holding a beat-up unidentifiable video.

"Yeah. Look at that thing, it's beat-up," I said joyfully.

"Don't put tapes like this into your TV anymore, you hear?"

"Yeah, I hear. Thanks for getting it fixed. Let's just toss it in the trash so it can't cause any more damage."

Little domestic episodes like this convinced me that I needed to get away from home and I was glad that I had college coming up. I applied for early admission to the University of Virginia. For my personal essay, I wrote passionately about my disease, as if I were speaking directly to the Ewing's sarcoma. After my mom edited my draft, she walked into my room with tears in her eyes. "Benjamin, I want you to know how inspirational this essay is," she said.

"Are you crying? Look, I don't mean half of that crap. I just wrote it so maybe it would help me get into UVA. I don't actually feel that way, so stop crying."

"I don't care, this means a lot to me."

"Whatever. I just want to get in."

I felt uncomfortable when others cried in my presence. And I hated showing sadness or vulnerability, especially in front of my parents. Sometimes it's necessary to shield them from the truth in order to protect them. That's why I don't answer my dad whenever he asks how I'm feeling. It's also why I don't tell them when health issues arise. In 2006, I broke my finger and didn't tell them for two months. By that point it was already healed, so there was nothing they could worry about.

I used to push my parents away in hopes that they would love me less. That way, they would feel less pain if something terrible happened to me. They always wanted to protect me from the cancer. But, I hated their protection. Some people advised me to open up to my parents and let them know exactly how I was feeling. I did not buy this. Instead I protected my parents by not letting them see my pain or hear me grouse. What if I whined about everything? Imagine how helpless my parents would feel. But even with my Superman façade, my parents stayed over-protective. For one thing, my dad wanted me to go to George Mason University. "That way, you can live at home."

"But, I don't want to live at home."

"I think you should. I went to Hofstra, and I lived at home. I just commuted an hour to and from Brooklyn."

My dad was concerned about me attending a college two hours away, but I was determined not to let cancer affect my decision. Actually, I was debating whether the hundred miles between Charlottesville and Manassas would be enough. UVA wait-listed me while I was accepted into William & Mary, Virginia Tech and James Madison University. Aunt Florence said she would pull some strings to get me into UVA. I still had to choose between the other three in case Aunt Florence came up empty-handed. My heart was leaning toward Tech because Jonathan was going there. My parents encouraged me to visit William & Mary for an open house, where I saw only six attractive girls out of the hundreds of potential students. That was what made me decide that it wasn't for me.

Just as I expected, Aunt Florence prevailed, and in the coolest way—my uncle's business partner talked to Virginia Governor Mark Warner, who had his people talk to UVA people. I was probably the last student accepted, receiving that delicate piece of mail in the middle of June.

I wasn't ready for college. Since I already lost an entire year of prime maturing time to cancer, how could I possibly manage? I would be away from home. I would have to befriend total strangers. And I would have

to explain all over again at least a hundred times why I wore a special shoe and had a massive scar that ends below my waistline. Not only did my scar come daringly close to my privates, half my pubic hair had been in the radiation field, so one side had no hair growth. When I mentioned it to my friends, I asked, "Do you sick bastards really want to see it? Fine." I pulled my pants down a couple of inches.

"Whoa shit, you weren't kidding!" Drew said. "Look at that. It's just a straight line down—one side hair, and the other side as smooth as a baby's ass."

"That's right, laugh it up."

Right then, one of my female crushes, Aaliyah Sandoval, walked through the door and saw the three of us staring down at my crotch. "What the hell are you guys doing?" she asked.

"Nothing," I said as I tugged my pants up.

Nonetheless, the next week I nervously asked Aaliyah to the senior prom. She turned me down. Nervous doesn't even describe how scared I was. Even though she rejected me, the fact that I even asked showed I was making progress.

In the sixth grade I had attended a school dance where an older girl said I looked like her uncle, and then she hoisted me up and spun me around. It was such a traumatizing experience that I began to avoid dancing the way I avoided salmon. At every dance thereafter I would craft an excuse why I couldn't attend, which usually revolved around Friday night Temple services that I didn't even go to. Songs like "Y.M.C.A." still struck fear in me because someone might expect me to start dancing. The cancer had gotten me this far, though. I could ask Aaliyah and survive her refusal because cancer had made all my other problems seem trivial. Still, I might call on the powers from my Super-Jew tee shirt which served me so well with the cancer to help me in social situations. I had gotten to the point where I had missed so much time and so many experiences that I just could not catch up entirely. Senior year almost felt like my high school

moved on and left me behind. There had not been a single picture or mention of me in my junior yearbook. I was a ghost. People would come up to me and ask: "Where have you been, I haven't seen you in forever?" Some of them did not even know that I had had cancer.

I surely left my mark in the senior yearbook. I was in the photographs for clubs I almost never participated in, like Quill and Scroll, which I wanted to be president of. Instead of being present at the election, I signed a paper that read, "Ben Rubenstein is running for president," and handed it to another member.

"Make sure they know I'm running," I told her. "And make sure I win." I didn't.

I was voted Parliamentarian of the Chess Club, even though I had no idea what that means and my final record there was 0-19. But since so many students who flooded the Chess Club photo weren't actually members of the club, the yearbook gave no mention of my official position. Drew, a non-member, claimed to be "Director of Pieces." I would have been pissed if they had printed that and not listed me as Parliamentarian.

At the end of the year, there was a ceremony for our graduating class. It was emceed by my teacher and former blood and platelet donor, Mr. Foley.

At the end of the ceremony, he read which college each of us was going to, as well as scholarships earned. One of the scholarships I earned was from the American Cancer Society. Not wanting to embarrass me, Mr. Foley hesitated before reading that one, unsure of whether or not he should even say it aloud. He did, but he blushed while he said it.

That was the approach most people took, based on my own lead—to move on as if cancer was a tiny roadblock from my past, not even deserving of mention. That's what I wanted to believe and the way I wanted others to perceive. I was a Super Man for having survived cancer without a flinch, not a wimp who got it in the first place. I didn't need to acknowledge that I was any less than normal or anything short of healthy. My supreme ability to fight cancer fueled my Super Man complex,

which further fueled my belief that I was invincible in every way. It was a cycle that I wholeheartedly embraced. It may be possible to leave the cancer itself in the dust the way I had attempted to but the experiences and memories, both positive and negative, would always be with me. They had helped shape the person I have become.

The governor of Virginia, Mark Warner—governor, senator, potential president, and reason I'm a Wahoo—spoke at my high school graduation. That night I went to Operation Graduation, an event meant to keep us graduates away from alcohol by locking us in the school until five in the morning. Rick needed to crap around midnight, so we tried unsuccessfully sneaking him into our Government teacher's room to poop on her desk. Later in the night, I was sitting at the blackjack table between Drew and Worm. I asked to sign Worm's yearbook. I opened the book to an empty space when I noticed Drew's shitty handwriting. His message read:

We have known each other since kindergarten, which is a shame. We make a great team. With Andy we are unstoppable. Remember that and to not get beat up by your roommate and you're good. I love you man.

With Andy we're unstoppable? Doesn't he mean with Andy and Ben we're unstoppable? This was written proof that cancer changes everything. I had suffered through fourteen chemo cycles, five weeks of radiation, removal of my left iliac wing and fifteen-and-a-half months of physical therapy. I had watched my friends have fun and grow closer to one another without me, but I had never held them back.

After treatment, I had tried my best to make everything go back to normal. I went through my senior year as if nothing had changed. But while I had been watching Matt and Charlie die and proving to myself that I could vanquish this tumor within me, my friends at Osbourn Park High School were getting on with their lives. They were not looking back or waiting for me to catch up.

My outlook on life stayed pretty positive as summer arrived. Then boom! I saw Dr. Wodajo for my standard six-month checkup. After

looking at my X-rays, he told me that the radiation had caused avascular necrosis, or bloodless death. The top of my femur, my hip joint and what remained of my left ilium were dying because they couldn't receive an adequate blood supply. It was then that I accepted the painful truth—I wouldn't run, jump or play sports again for the rest of my life. The closest I'll ever come to physical competition is a rousing game of Ping-Pong. If only I was as easy to please as Forrest Gump.

The assurance Dr. Merlin had given me—that eventually I would play tackle football—was false. Either he was bullshitting me, or he had had to remove more bone than he had expected. I wasn't mad at him, though. If anything, his prognosis had motivated me to work harder. That afternoon, I made it my lifelong goal to rehab my hip; to get it as close to normal as humanly, or in my case superhumanly, possible.

My inability to engage in physical activity turned out to be my most life-changing sacrifice. I can't watch a sporting event without wishing I could play. I can't walk anywhere without being conscious of my gait. Above all, I cannot stop living in the past, revising history in my head so that I wouldn't have physical limitations. Sometimes I wonder if seeing a doctor sooner would have changed anything. Or had not continued playing tennis when the pain started. I have to remind myself that my cancer had not spread, and that I am still alive. Sometimes in the summer, when I wear shorts and sneakers, I look down at my calves and ankles. This part of my body didn't change much from when I was sixteen. That's when I can picture myself as Pre-Cancer Ben.

Several times each year for six years, I dreamed that I ran as hard as I could to nowhere in particular. I would have a smile on my face when I woke up in the morning because in the dream I had felt the familiar rush of excitement and adrenaline of physical performance. Once those dreams ended, I started dreaming that I am playing baseball one-on-one against Jeff Kent, a onetime Major League Baseball MVP. I throw heat and he hits a high, deep pop-up. I run past the infield to the grass, pick

up speed and sprint, my legs moving instinctively. Then I halt and watch as the ball drops in front of me. Eight years and many runs later, I finally understand this dream.

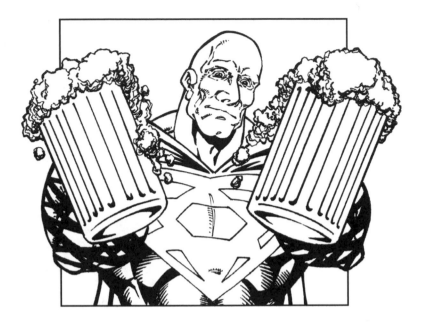

Chapter 6
ROUND TWO

When I arrived at UVA as a freshman, I lived in Humphreys which the guys called The Hump. The resident advisor there gathered us around to play Break The Ice. Each person tells three things about himself—two true and one false. I had planned on saying, "I have a brother at Virginia Tech, my parents are midgets and, oh yeah, I had cancer." When the moment came, though, I could not bring myself to mention my cancer. Instead, I stated that I loved the Redskins.

There was no getting around my fifteen-inch scar, though, so when he asked, I told my roommate Derek Miller. Derek was one of the few people who seemed interested in my past. After I mentioned my Make-A-Wish gift, he said, "You should bring your TV to school. It would take up our entire room, but it would be worth it. I'm willing to sleep

on the hallway floor."

Word got around after that and I always wondered who told whom, who else knew. I wanted everyone to know but my No Complaining rule prohibited me from telling people. So I started walking around shirtless to provoke inquiries. Some guys glanced away, while others just didn't notice. That rule, which basically governed my life, held me back in terms of making friends in college. But more importantly, the rule— not talking about cancer and never complaining about anything—was part of why I felt so unique and strong, and anything else that created the cancer-slaying Super Man that I became. If I were to abolish the rule, then I would also be letting go of that force within me. It wasn't even a choice; because I could not imagine my life without that rule.

I found myself hanging out with Nick and Tim, friends from high school, more than the guys from my dorm. I used the old friends so I would not have to meet new people. Even though I had felt a little left out my senior year, once I got to Charlottesville I clung to that crowd. I felt like the guys I knew already had gone through cancer with me simply because we were at school together during my treatment. It didn't matter how close we were in high school or even if we were friends at all. They were there, they saw me survive and that was enough for me to feel comfortable around them. Social insecurity is normal among cancer survivors, but I found it disappointing when it happened to me. I wanted to fit in and be myself, but my medical past formed an insurmountable barrier.

My hallmates were always playing Four-Square. Whenever they asked me to join, I would say, "I don't play kids' games." They probably assumed I didn't like playing sports. I wanted to tell them that at one point in my life, not too long ago, I was quick with a sweet jump shot and a decent serve. But I could not prove it. I had lost the jump and the serve. Rather than explain, I lived with them thinking of me as an unathletic nerd.

When I went home for breaks, my great friends from high school were moving in new directions. Andy and Drew had joined fraternities—Andy at Clemson, and Drew at Virginia Tech. That was all they discussed—their frat brothers, the funny hazing methods and which sororities had the prettiest girls. Andy and Drew were having the time of their lives, but I was not. Don't get me wrong—I enjoyed college. I loved the freedom and making my own decisions. It was tough enough being separated at different colleges, but now they were in a new world. I was stuck in the past. Some of us in the hall would play *Halo* on Xbox for hours, even skipping classes. I brought my PS2, and at the end of October, I purchased *Grand Theft Auto: Vice City*. For the next few weeks, Derek and I left our door unlocked because there was always somebody in there playing.

The Hump was acclaimed across the campus for the two star athletes, two future senators, real-life nephew to Uncle Phil from *The Fresh Prince of Bel-Air* and potential serial killer living there. I was never going to be a jock again, but at least I could hang with them in The Hump. D'Brickashaw Ferguson, UVA's stud offensive lineman who went on to play for the New York Jets, lived in the basement. He and I were like brothers, and by that I mean we nodded to each other in passing. Ryan Zimmerman, the fourth overall pick in the 2005 baseball draft and an All-Star for the Washington Nationals, was the only person to ever beat me at *Tiger Woods PGA Tour 2003*.

I was overwhelmed by the number of pretty girls on campus. They were everywhere. When it was warm, they sunbathed on the quad. Growing out of my extreme shyness around girls has been a gradual process but that first semester I did chat with one of the most beautiful girls I have seen—after Lily, of course. I even invited her to a party. "No thanks," she said. I had been rejected in high school, so I was used to "no." I always believed that things would work out at a later date. It was only years later, when I became aware that she (as well as Lily) was engaged to

someone not me that I saw my dreams shatter. I kept trying to get girls. I decided to try advancing a friendship into seduction. In my most ballsy move ever, I told a friend I had a crush on her.

"Really? I had no idea," she said.

"Yeah, for like two months now."

"Wow. Thanks."

Not exactly the response I was looking for. But I was not able to get any further. My tongue was tied. The next day, I e-mailed her, "Sorry about yesterday. That's something that nobody should ever do sober."

Before college I was always sober. I hadn't had much experience with alcohol; the first time I drank was in Israel with Jonathan when I was sixteen. He bought a bottle of vodka and took long, gulping swigs. He made it look so easy that I didn't think I needed a chaser. I grabbed the bottle, chugged, then stared blankly across the room at a hot girl before coughing uncontrollably. "That shit burns!"

I knew that college guys did things I had never done at home: drinking, fighting and getting laid. So as soon as I could get in, I started going to bars. I began to understand why alcohol is called the solvent of the superego. I had never been in a fight, but after a few drinks, I found myself wanting to start one. I never followed the impulse for fear of shattering my hip but my imagination wandered to a daydream where I would start a fight, take a punch or two, back out and then let my friends take over the fight for me. Some of the guys I knew would have killed for me, and I kind of wanted to witness it.

I got pretty suave at the bar chat. After the first weeks in The Hump, I had gotten comfortable pulling the cancer card though in a normal state of consciousness, I rarely did. Sometimes when I was intoxicated, though, it could become a prime topic of conversation. Originally, I had expected that girls would give the "Aww" squeal and melt in the palm of my hand when I told them about the cancer. It didn't work that way: girls were taken aback, embarrassed, awed. It was a complete

conversation stopper. Yet guys would respond drunkenly with enthusiasm, delivering incoherent speeches on how much they admired me for surviving.

Once, a conversation with a pretty girl was going well until I said, "I'd offer to buy you a drink, but I see you are holding one in your hand right now."

"Uh, yeah. Good observation," she said.

"Thank you."

Perhaps I should have walked away at that point but I had an idea that if I kept drinking I could keep talking and if I could keep talking, I might get the girl. I persisted until I could not think of anything else to say. There was a long pause, and then I ended it with, "I'm going to see what my buddy's up to. It's nice to meet you. My name is Ben, but I don't think you gave me yours."

"Yes I did. It's Gayle."

"Oh. Well, see you later."

I did see her the following week and approached her again. "I remember you from last week. And I know your name this time. It's Kayle."

"No, it's not. It's Gayle."

End of that conversation right there.

That terrifying sixth grade dance many years earlier undermined my confidence on the dance floor. But one night, I was so intoxicated that I broke my No Dancing rule. I settled in one section of the bar and commenced to dance by myself. Drew sat next to me, laughing at me. After several seconds of this disgrace, a very tall girl got behind me. With my back to her, I signaled to Drew that she was huge by lifting my arm in the air and moving my hand up and down like an elevator.

"She's a monster," I whispered to Drew. I hoped she didn't hear me, or notice me waving my hand.

I moved to the right. She moved with me.

I moved to the left. She moved with me.

I moved right again. She moved with me again.

Then, she tapped me on the shoulder. "No, I'm actually just trying to get by," she said.

It didn't surprise me that I was a flop with girls in college because I had gotten off to a bad start senior year. The week following my high school graduation was Beach Week when everybody went to Myrtle Beach to get drunk. The cancer had inhibited the development of my drinking career. I was not sure it was okay to drink alcohol, so I secretly asked my nurse. "I drank when I was your age, so I'm not going to give you the 'don't drink' speech. Just go slow."

When Andy and I arrived at Myrtle, I immediately asked if he wanted to start drinking. "Yeah, man. Give me a few minutes."

I couldn't wait. I filled a cup with Bacardi and Sierra Mist. After guzzling it, I poured another, angry that I didn't feel any different. Andy walked in as I poured my third cup. "You started without me?"

"I couldn't wait for your lazy ass. It's drinking time!"

Are you drunk already?"

"No. At least, I don't think so."

I didn't know the difference between having a buzz and being drunk. I liquored up so fast that I must have skipped the buzzing step altogether. I hit the streets and made my rounds to my friends' houses, drinking beer all along the way. Places to go, people to see.

As the night rolled on, I got more and more drunk. I didn't know what my limit was, and frankly I didn't care—I was having the time of my life. I had long, deep conversations with anyone who would listen, and thus became known as The Philosophical Drunk. I had my conversation with my friend Terry around midnight. She was drinking a lemonade/vodka concoction and no longer wanted it. "I'll take it," I told her.

That got me really fucked-up. I saw triple everything, which reminded me of *Rocky IV.* "Hit the one in the middle, Benjy, hit the one

in the middle," I repeated to myself. I blacked out after that, and remembered later that Terry walked me back to my beach house. She placed a trash can next to me in case I needed to vomit. "Oh gosh," I said. "I hate vomiting. I did enough of it in the hospital last year."

"I know, Ben. I'm sorry," Terry said.

The next morning battling the worst hangover, I eventually gathered the balls to gag myself. Worm woke up to the sound of my vomit. "That's the second time I have heard you puke," he said accusingly.

Two nights later, we went to a strip club. I climbed in the back of my friend's SUV, when Rick, who was sitting right next to me, threw up into a Solo cup. It didn't hold all his vomit, which overflowed onto the carpet. That's the last thing I remember of that night.

When I saw Bently the following afternoon, he was laughing uncontrollably. "What the hell are you laughing at?" I asked.

"Oh Benjy, Benjy, Benjy. Tell me you remember what happened last night?"

"I remember getting in the car to go to the strip club. I remember Rick puking in that cup. That's all. What happened?"

"When we got there, you were completely zoned out. We paid for you to get a lap dance. When you were done, the stripper came back to talk to us. She said that you passed out during the lap dance and she asked us if you were all right. She said that she'd never had that happen to her."

"No way. Are you lying?"

"No. We all just started cracking up."

"I'm never going to a strip club again." That would have been the easy way to hook up with a woman but strip clubs were obviously not going to work for me. Alcohol didn't deliver me from my inhibitions as it did for my friends who gradually became different people while drinking. I was pretty much the same drunk as not drunk. I wished I could be transformed by alcohol and become someone else, as they did. Instead of being the perpetual nice guy, I would like to give girls a hard time

like Worm always did. Strangely, drunken girls seem to gravitate towards sarcastic louts.

Probably because of the chemo, my body wouldn't allow me to drink as much as I wanted to. That's probably a good thing. Unlike some of my friends who have iron stomachs, I puked most weekends during my first semester at UVA.

I wanted to perform the rite of passage that every college kid is entitled to: have lots of strange, casual sex. Movies and statistics show how normal it is. It seemed so simple: go to a party hammered, grind on a girl on the dance floor and take her back to the dorm. This was an unlikely scenario for me to begin with. I was short and reserved, while the guys who got the girls were tall and aggressive. I felt that I could not attract a girl without my prized curly hair.

I resigned myself to the fact that it was never going to happen. Not getting laid meant I was inadequate, flawed and unwanted. As I tried attending more and more parties, I began to wonder if not even being acknowledged by the girls meant I didn't exist. If Ben goes to a party and nobody notices him, was he really there? By the time I got to the first anniversary of finishing cancer treatment I had given up on girls and focused on getting drunk.

I wanted to celebrate the one-year anniversary of finishing cancer treatment the right way—get hammertime, shitfaced, blitzbashed, fucked-up drunk. If I didn't puke, then I hadn't drunk enough. A friend from high school joined me as we celebrated the First Annual Cancer Raping Celebration Drunkfest (CRCD).

Over the course of two hours, we finished a fifth of Ice 101 Peppermint Schnapps, then headed to the frat houses. I remember little of what happened the rest of the night. I can't say it was enjoyable, but I was thrilled with how wasted I got—puking for an hour, including on a frat house floor and some girl's shoes. Back at The Hump, I walked into my room where some of my hallmates were playing PS2. I braced myself

on the wall, looked at them, and prepared to say something important…"I have to brush my teeth!"

I began to wonder what I was doing at UVA. I refused to sacrifice going to the gym, sleeping or watching TV just to study. My goal had become dropping my GPA to just above an academic warning. A warning came at 1.8. I got a 1.97. I was doing just well enough not to be a fuck-up. I began to question my own intelligence. Did I even belong at UVA? I couldn't fight, fuck or handle alcohol—was there anything I could do during college? Well, there was always football.

After Thanksgiving, it was time to show Jonathan and Drew that UVA was better than Tech during our annual rivalry game. At Jonathan's tailgate, he and his friends were talking shit.

"Face it, Benjamin," Jonathan said, "Lee Suggs and Kevin Jones are going to run for five touchdowns each and UVA will lose 70-0."

"We'll see about that."

"So how do you like Tech so far?"

"It's pretty cool. I like how much energy your fans have; definitely more than at a UVA game."

"You should have come here. Just wait until we get inside the stadium. It's going to be a sea of maroon and orange."

Jonathan proceeded to mock my school's tradition of wearing a shirt and tie to football games. (I'm proud to say I never participated in that tradition.) It was bitter cold with heavy snow and strong winds. The weather made it nearly impossible to throw, as indicated by Matt Schaub's forty-three total passing yards. The Hokies won 21-9 in a closer game than the score indicated. My hands were nearly frozen, so it was hard to care that much.

Afterwards, we got drunk at Jonathan's frat house, where he was the house manager and would soon win his fraternity's Brother of the Year Award. I loved hanging out with Jonathan, but it was weird being his peer instead of his younger brother. I began to wonder when he lost

his virginity, or how many times he'd smoked weed, or if he'd tried my favorite drug, oxycodone. I wondered how many girlfriends he'd had. I realized I really didn't know much about him at all.

Winter break was like old times, only with alcohol. I spent many nights at Brent Birdsall's house drinking Bud Diesel. In the seventh grade, Birdsall and I had co-founded The Posse, and had recruited our ten best friends to be in it. We'd even had a secret hand signal which we would flash whenever we'd passed each other in the halls at school. Later in the year, we had ended The Posse when we'd realized how lame it was.

Birdsall and I started talking about my eighteen-month post-treatment checkup, scheduled for the following day, which consisted only of a physical, blood work, and a chest X-ray. "What kind of appointment do you have tomorrow?" Birdsall asked.

"It's nothing, just a standard visit."

"I pray for you every time you tell me you're going to the doctor."

"Thanks, dude, but really, this is a piece of cake."

"I pray anyway. You know I cried when you told me you got cancer."

"Are you serious? Damn man, even I didn't cry."

"I just went to my room that night and started crying. You're such a good guy; I couldn't believe that happened to you."

"Thanks man, but I don't need the prayers. I'm doing really well." I said this because everyone commented on how healthy I looked, how well I was doing. Birdsall could save his prayers because my appointment the next day was just following protocol, more of a social visit than anything else.

The eighteen-month restaging, exactly two years after my hip surgery, was the first time I had seen my hospital friends since the summer. Christine had gone to UVA so I wanted to fill her in on my experiences there. The docs expected that I would remain healthy and I felt just as strong as I did when I was sixteen.

I was disappointed to learn that Lisa no longer worked as a nurse in the pediatric cancer unit, but had moved to Research on the same floor. I guessed that she could no longer cope with the sadness of getting to know Sick Kids, only to watch them suffer and die. Back when I was getting treatment, Lisa had asked me if I wanted to be a doctor when I grew up. "Are you going into medicine? Or maybe try to cure cancer?"

"Yeah, right. Once I finish treatment, I'm going to walk away and never look back at this or any other hospital."

Christine's physical exam was of course nonchalant. Everything was normal, except for some bruises which neither of us heeded. Before leaving, I asked if my blood results were in the computer.

"I don't think so, but let me check."

Fifteen seconds and several mouse clicks later, Christine said with a surprised tone, "They have you red-flagged."

"What does 'red-flagged' mean?"

"Your platelets are 24 thousand."

Boom! It was the most common of blood tests that changed everything. My bone marrow was dying without my even knowing it. No clue, no idea, never crossed my mind, impossible. IMPOSSIBLE. The words "bone marrow transplant" flashed in my head like a lightning storm. I knew Round II had begun, and my life was about to change again.

"24 thousand? Oh, my God. Normally, I'm way over 200 thousand. What does this mean?"

"Ben, let's not jump to conclusions. This could be a fluke. Don't worry about this just yet. We'll take your blood again, and hopefully we'll see that it was a false reading."

I knew it wasn't a fluke. I had just remembered that I had been bruising for at least a month now, an obvious sign of low platelets. I was mentally preparing myself for battle with my second severe illness. I was the self-proclaimed Greatest Cancer Patient Ever and I had to live up to my reputation.

Telling my dad in the waiting room was nauseating. "What does that mean?" he asked me.

"Nothing, yet. They're going to recheck my blood to see if this was a screw-up," I said as cheerfully as possible.

The two of us waited, jittery and quiet. I listened to 3 Doors Down's *"Away from the Sun"* on my CD player, hoping it would displace me from reality. About an hour later, Christine came out to tell me the platelets were not a fluke, that they were 24 thousand, an extremely low number for a cancer survivor in remission. She took me and my dad into a side room, the exact same room where I was told I had Ewing's sarcoma. The exact same fucking room where my parents signed documents that suggested, "Benjamin can die this many different ways," over two years earlier. Give me some privacy there, and I'll make Ron Artest at The Malice at the Palace look like a chump.

Gathered around the table were my dad, Christine, Dr. Levy who was chief of the pediatric oncology branch, and myself. Christine, who normally had the ability to inspirit a damp sponge, looked lifeless. My dad struggled to keep from shedding tears the entire meeting, but I stayed relatively calm, for myself and for him. "Now that we know this is real, what is causing my low platelets?" I asked.

"We don't know," the chief said. "There are so many possibilities. We don't need to discuss them now."

"Wait, wait a second," my dad said. "He's been going to school, he's been healthy, I don't understand."

"That's great that he's been doing so well," Christine said. "If he were really sick then we'd be more concerned. But we do need to figure out what is causing his low platelets. We'll schedule Ben for a bone marrow biopsy on Monday."

I said "Okay," and took a long pause. "Am I going to need a bone marrow transplant?"

"Please say no, please say no." I thought the whole time.

"That would be a long ways down the road because we don't even know what's causing your low platelets," Chief Levy said.

My dad spoke, but had trouble putting syllables together. "Wait, wait, wait…what…what do you mean 'bone marrow transplant'?"

"That would only be done if this is a certain disease," the chief reiterated. "This could be nothing, or it could be some kind of disease. Right now we have no idea."

My dad didn't have the foresight the rest of us did, and nobody had the heart to tell him. I offered to drive us home, but my dad refused, as if guiding the Big Red Box could somehow incite my bone marrow to start working again. We stopped to eat at Roy Rogers, not because we were hungry, but because that had been our plan.

I have had terrible ear problems my whole life—infections, tubes, surgeries, the threat of deafness and unbearable pain. My dad once had to hold me down as my ENT cauterized my eardrum and sucked out the pus that seemed could only come from my brain. My horrifying screams were heard from the waiting room. I would dread visiting my ENT days in advance. But after each visit, my dad treated me to Roy Rogers.

"Why did you say bone marrow transplant?" my dad asked as we slowly ate out sandwiches.

"That's what might need to be done."

"Yeah but, why did you say that?"

"Never mind. Don't worry about it."

My dad couldn't understand. For the next few years, Roy's roast beef tasted like fear to me.

When we got home, my mom asked how things went, and I gave her the sugar-coated version. Still, seeing her face and say, "Oh dear God," broke my heart. I left our conversation and headed to the basement where my fifty-three inch TV could make me feel safe. She called Chief Levy.

"What did he tell you?" I asked.

"He said that 'lightning doesn't strike twice,' and the chances of this being leukemia are small."

I had assumed my bone marrow was failing. It hadn't occurred to me that this might actually be cancer again. That suggestion made me dizzy and seasick, like my couch dropped from under me. If I have to go through fourteen more cycles of chemo…No. I can't do it. I won't do it.

When Jonathan got home, I gave him the version with extra frosting. Jonathan, my dad and I played darts before dinner, which helped distract me. It helped so much that I played every day I was home for the next three months.

Later that night, I called Drew. "Hey Drew, what are you doing?"

"I'm playing *Vice City*. I can't get past this stupid mission."

"Can I come over? I have something to tell you."

"Yeah, sure."

I went down to his basement, where I found him playing *Grand Theft Auto*. "Have you beaten this mission, yet?" he asked. "I can't do it."

"Yeah, I'll beat it for you in a second. I had my year-and-a-half check-up at NIH, today. It turns out that my platelets are really low."

"What does that mean?"

"It could mean a lot of things. Nobody knows yet."

"Damn."

There wasn't much else to say about it. I beat the mission for him, and then we talked about school. I later told my roommate, Derek, I wouldn't make it back for a week or two. I'll never forget the message Birdsall left on my answering machine after he heard. "My mom just told me. I can't believe it. I don't know what to say. Tell me if there's anything I can do." That was probably the feeling most people close to me felt—helplessness and disbelief.

My parents and I arrived early at NIH three days later for my bone marrow biopsy. My platelets were twenty-one thousand and I needed a transfusion before the procedure. They dropped by three thousand in

three days. What's happening to me?

While waiting, Christine told me I would receive conscious sedation for the biopsy—a combination of Versed and fentanyl. "Versed is like Valium, and fentanyl is like morphine, but they're both ten times stronger and short-acting," she said. I later read that fentanyl is estimated to be fifty to one hundred times more potent than morphine. Death is so swift that some addicts have died with the needle still in their vein. Christine had me lie on my stomach and drop my pants, and then gave me the IV. The two drugs hit hard, and it was wonderful. "I'm ridiculously high right now," I remember telling her.

I was told I wouldn't recall anything, though I do remember talking the whole time and having Christine show me what the marrow looks like (red Jell-O). Christine claimed that I talked about partying at school, and I couldn't tell if she was joking.

The biopsy was not only easy, but actually enjoyable, which made me feel hopeful. Christine and Chief Levy made me feel safe. "You will be back at UVA, I promise," the chief said to me.

One week later, Christine said that the biopsy showed no sign of leukemia, my biggest concern. Other than having fewer cells than normal, the results were ordinary. Christine immediately scheduled me for a second biopsy, which was much less nerve-racking than the first. I was even looking forward to it because of the high. After that was over, Christine encouraged me to return to school. "I think it'll be good for you to be around your friends. I'm sure they're all worried about you."

I knew Derek would have told my hallmates about my old cancer, as well as the new scare, so I was nervous the first time back. I had to calm myself down once I neared campus. The thought of being looked at once again as the Sick Kid made me want to puke. Can't they see I'm a Super Man? My hallmates were outside playing football when I arrived and chanted "Ru-ben-stein" when I approached. They were supportive in a subtle way. I didn't want anybody's pity, and I'm certain they knew that.

A few of us watched Super Bowl XXXVII with the Oakland Raiders vs. the Tampa Bay Buccaneers in my room. Drew grew up a Raiders fan, so if they won, I knew I would never hear the end of it. Fortunately, Tampa Bay smoked them, 48-21. I called Drew when the game was over, and was greeted with, "Shut the hell up!"

"Good game," I said laughing.

"I don't want to talk about it. Anyway, how did the Redskins do this year?"

"They didn't lose in the Super Bowl, I can tell you that much."

I harassed Drew some more, and then called Worm. We talked about how great the outcome of the game was and how promising the Redskins were going to be next season. The only way to relieve the sadness of one NFL season ending is to talk about the next one.

The next morning I woke up hearing myself shouting, "Get me a tissue!"

"Shit man, you got a lot of blood there," Derek said.

I had felt an itch on my nose as I was waking up. I suppressed it with my navy blue sweatshirt, and looked down in horror as I saw red fluid covering the end of my sleeve.

"What do I do? I have never had a nosebleed."

"Pinch your nose with the tissue and tilt your head back."

It didn't work. I was going through tissues like toilet paper after eating bad Chinese food. Each tissue was soaked in blood, and there was no stopping the downpour. I called NIH and asked to speak with the doctor on call. "Hey Ben, this is Dr. Springs."

"How's it going, Dr. Springs? Long time no see. I was sitting here when suddenly my nose started bleeding. I think my platelets may be low."

"How fast is the blood coming out?"

"Pretty fast. I'm mowing through my box of tissues."

"Okay. Do you know the phone number to the Hematology/Oncology clinic down there at UVA?"

"Shit, I don't know."

"That's okay. Do you have access to a car?"

"Yeah, my car is right outside my dorm."

"Go to the ER and give them your name. I'm going to call them and tell them you're coming, so they'll be expecting you."

As I hung up, Derek was standing in the doorway with his sandals on and my keys in his hand. "Benjy, you ready to go?"

Derek dropped me off at the ER, and left to go park my car. My bleeding finally slowed while I was in the waiting room. A nurse took me to a patient room and inserted an IV to take blood. "The results will take an hour. Then we'll get you some platelets." My platelet transfusion couldn't come soon enough—the blood loss from my nose was replaced by an IV. It was coating my arm red, all the way down to my hand.

I had just finished cleaning my arm in the bathroom when Derek returned. "Hey bud, did the bleeding stop yet?"

"Almost. She just took my blood, so it'll take an hour before I get the results. You can head back if you want."

"Nah, that's alright. If I go back, then I have to do work. I'd much rather just watch TV here."

"Thanks man."

When I first met Derek I didn't like him much and had trouble getting used to his quirks. He always listened to the same alternative rock songs. He talked a lot and had a southern accent. He went to sleep early. He was jumpy, like he had ADD or something. He didn't wash his hands after going to the bathroom. And he always said the phrase, "I'm going to hit the sack." Over time, he grew on me. After that night, I considered Derek my good friend.

I was almost certain I wouldn't finish the semester, so I skipped most classes. I also had restrictions on exercising. And the one time I partied, I was terrified the alcohol would cause internal bleeding because of my low platelets. Derek and I used to leave our door open, but I began clos-

ing it because I felt like such a loser when people passed by several times, and I was still playing *Grand Theft Auto: Vice City*. My only accomplishment was creating a compilation CD of the best *Vice City* songs and copying it for my hallmates. There was some kickass eighties music on that game.

My bone marrow was dying so fast it was scary. Along with my platelets, my red blood cells were also disappearing. Within weeks of finding out there was a problem, I was already getting blood and platelet transfusions regularly. If I wasn't in my dorm room playing PS2, I was probably hooked up to an IV at the UVA Hematology/Oncology clinic.

I realized that I was wasting my parents' money by staying at school. Fortunately, they could still get a refund on my tuition. I met with the dean to discuss my withdrawal. He wished me luck and assured me that when I was ready, UVA would be waiting. I turned in my student ID, and that was it. I was no longer a student at the University of Virginia.

It was embarrassing how I handled my departure. Terry said, "I would have made my hallmates throw a huge party for me." Instead, I sent this e-mail:

> Date: Wednesday, February 26, 2003
>
> To: my 22 hallmates
>
> I will not be coming back here after spring break. I'm leaving for good. I will be back next year. I'll still have instant messenger if you want to keep in touch. I don't give a fuck if you ask me what the problem is, you just won't hear me bring it up much. Peace out fuckers.

After Derek and others loaded my belongings into the Big Red Box, I went back to my room one more time. "It looks so pathetic," I said.

"I know," Derek said. "I think I'm going to put the TV on your old desk. And your bed could become like a couch."

"That's a good idea."

It was like I had never been there to begin with. The room looked so empty, mostly because Derek barely owned anything. Other than a single semester and a few new friends, there wasn't much proof I was ever a Wahoo. Maybe I should have brought my fifty-three inch sweetheart after all, and then left it behind—now that would have been a worthy legacy.

NIH did not possess the technology to diagnose my problem, so they referred me to Johns Hopkins Hospital, one of the best hospitals in the world. It stood out in its run-down East Baltimore neighborhood. The brand-new Weinberg Building, a 380 thousand-square-foot marvel, was where we came in. The building was so high-tech that patients received a bright orange card that digitally contained all of his or her information. We were scheduled to meet with Dr. Ford, head of the adult bone marrow transplant program at Hopkins. Dr. Ford was a big deal. I was impressed with how approachable Dr. Ford was, despite his huge reputation. He knew I had one of two diseases—aplastic anemia or myelodysplatic syndrome, also known as myelodysplasia. A bone marrow transplant is the only known cure for these diseases.

If I had aplastic anemia, then the recovery time would be forty-two days. I would stay in the hospital for half the time, and move to an apartment nearby for the rest. According to Dr. Ford, the survival rate for aplastic anemia, treated at Hopkins, is a whopping eighty-five percent, much higher than the rate for Ewing's sarcoma which I had already weathered. First they would give me chemo, specifically the drug Cytoxan, to destroy my existing bone marrow. I had been given that drug two years before so that wasn't so bad. I knew I could manage it. "Yes, but this would be ten times more toxic than for your previous cancer," Dr. Ford explained when I told him.

If I had myelodysplasia, I would receive a similar chemo regimen, but my recovery would take twice as long, and my chance of survival was

much less than eight-five percent. If left untreated, myelodysplasia can turn into full-blown leukemia. That's why it used to be termed "pre-leukemia," but according to the American Cancer Society, myelodysplasia is now classified as a form of cancer. I was happy that Dr. Ford guessed I had aplastic anemia.

Whichever disease I had, it was almost certainly caused by the Cytoxan chemotherapy I received for Ewing's sarcoma. The same chemical that destroyed my first life-threatening illness caused a second life-threatening illness. Ironically, it would also be the cure. Although this happened to about one in a hundred cancer patients, nobody had bothered to warn me this was a possibility.

After talking to Dr. Ford, I scheduled a bone marrow biopsy at Hopkins on Valentine's Day to determine which disease I had. "Dear God, please give me aplastic anemia," I prayed. It was the third consecutive year that cupid struck me with a trip to the hospital—on Valentine's Day in 2001 I began Cycle Six, and in 2002 I was hospitalized with the shingles. Now I was undergoing a bone marrow biopsy.

When Dr. Ford told me that I would be getting another biopsy, I explained to him that at NIH, they had difficulty finding the marrow. My hip was basically empty.

"Not to worry. Dr. Morgan here has performed hundreds of biopsies, and she's never failed to get a marrow sample. If she can't retrieve marrow from your hip, then we can always get it from your sternum."

"My what?"

"Your breastbone. It's very safe. We extract it from the sternum routinely."

"Could you try my hip first? I'd rather not have a needle in my chest."

When my blood and platelet transfusions were complete, my dad left the room and two people entered—Dr. Ford's sidekick, Dr. Connors, and the marrow-sucker, Dr. Morgan. "Dr. Ford said you were exceptional at biopsies," I said to her.

"Is that right? Well, I've done this quite a few times."

"There isn't much marrow to suck out."

"That shouldn't be a problem."

Once the Versed and fentanyl hit me, I escaped to my happy place. I didn't care that this woman was about to jab a thick needle through my bone to fetch what remained of my red Jell-O. She set the needle in the correct place, and the sucking commenced. After several minutes, she withdrew the needle, unable to collect any marrow, just as I had expected.

I rolled over onto my back, hoping the next needle through my chest wouldn't stab my heart or lungs. I took shallow breaths and placed a towel over my eyes. I couldn't watch.

Afraid to disappoint Dr. Ford, she had to report that two attempts failed. That's when Dr. Ford appeared in my room. "Hey, Dr. Ford. I didn't think I'd see you today," I said.

"Well Ben, I guess you were right about that marrow."

He told the nurse to pump me up with more drugs, and had me roll back onto my stomach for my third biopsy in an hour. Theoretically, there had to be some marrow left, and Dr. Ford was determined to unearth it. He pushed and pulled on the syringe in an attempt to suck every last drop out of the largest marrow-producing bone in my body. After several minutes of torture, he gathered the smallest amount of Jell-O to finally determine the demise of my once-indestructible bone marrow. The waiting game had begun. Did I have myelodysplasia or aplastic anemia? I prayed for the anemia.

The results arrived almost two weeks later. Dr. Ford's prediction was wrong. "We got a message from Hopkins—you have myelodys...however you say it," my dad said.

"Myelodysplasia. I guess I need a bone marrow transplant, huh?

"Yeah."

Chief Levy had said to my mom, "Lightning doesn't strike twice in

the same place" but that's bullshit: Studies with high-speed cameras have shown that most lightning flashes are multiple events, consisting of as many as forty-two main strokes, each of which is preceded by a leader stroke. I was getting tired of doctors telling me the statistically more probable option and having to deal with the dreaded alternative once the test results came in. Had they really believed the worst could not happen? How many more strikes would I have to endure?

Once the diagnosis was made, Dr. Ford's sidekick Dr. Connors took over my treatment. On my dad's fifty-eighth birthday, I met with him and my family to learn more about my cancer. His office was barely large enough to accommodate the five of us. Dr. Connors took a direct approach with us.

I had myelodysplasia monosomy 7, an acquired genetic abnormality of the bone marrow in which the seventh chromosome had mutated. There were three options. The first was to do nothing. "If you do nothing, then you'll eventually get leukemia. If that happens, your chances of survival are greatly decreased," he said.

"By how much? If I choose to do nothing, what's the likelihood that I'll develop leukemia?"

"Nothing is for sure, but I would have to say ninety-nine percent."

The second choice was drug treatment that would extend my life, but not cure my disease. "You would live for another three to four years. How old are you, Ben?"

"Nineteen."

"Well, I don't think you want to plan on living only until you're twenty-two or twenty-three years old. I'm sure you hope to live at least into your sixties. Am I right?"

"Yes."

"In that case, you have a third option that is proven to cure your disease: a bone marrow transplant."

The best scenario would be if Jonathan were a perfect bone marrow

donor match, which had a twenty-five percent probability of taking. Unfortunately, he wasn't. My mom had extended family members tested to see if they were a match. "That's fine, but the only person who really has a chance of being a match is his brother," Dr. Connors said. "If you choose somebody randomly, he'd have less than a .0001% chance of being Ben's exact match. There are some people who have been searching for an unrelated donor match for years."

I asked what my chance of surviving a bone marrow transplant was. Without hesitating he said, "The universal number is thirty percent." Thirty percent chance of living. Seventy percent chance of dying. My heart skipped a few beats.

At the end of the meeting, he said I would probably experience depression. "What do you mean? I don't get depressed," I said.

"Almost all patients do. A transplant is difficult. Don't expect to breeze through it." When I asked if the hospital had cable television, he looked at me like I was crazy. I guess he didn't know that ESPN was better than Prozac.

After the meeting Jonathan helped to keep me positive. Many elderly people get myelodysplasia, so we immediately bumped my survival chance up to fifty percent. And since I was a Super Man, I rounded it up to eighty percent. An eighty percent chance of survival for a normal person would mean a sure thing for me. In a flash of mental mathematics, I transformed my thirty percent chance of survival to nearly a hundred percent certainty. I was developing my own statistics.

Call it superstitious or psychotic if you'd like. I did not care what the official statistic was. My arrogance made me believe I would survive, which then helped me to actually survive. It is times like that I wouldn't give up my Super Man complex for all the friends, girls, money and success in the world.

I ate dinner with my family at ESPN Zone in Baltimore. We arrived just in time to see my two favorite sports shows, *Around the Horn* and

Pardon the Interruption. We sat in a circular booth in perfect view of the projection screen. I switched between looking at the huge screen and the smaller LCD attached to our table. I ordered the chicken cheese steak and fries, the same as Jonathan, and it was one of the most enjoyable meals I have ever had. I was thrilled about my upcoming journey, and savored my high chance of survival along with my fries.

Was I nuts? Hell yes. But I'm as proud of that nineteen-year-old Ben as anyone could be. Who else could manipulate such negative news into positive? I doubt I could duplicate that feat now.

I wanted to stay at Hopkins. There were three other top transplant centers my mom had researched: Children's Hospital of Wisconsin in Milwaukee; the University of Washington Medical Center in Seattle; and the University of Minnesota Medical Center in Minneapolis.

"Those other places are so far away, and Hopkins is a great hospital," I said.

Jonathan agreed. My dad also wanted me to stay at Hopkins as well, but I suspect that was influenced by his intense fear of flying. As far as finding a donor, I heard a story of a boy with five other siblings, and three of them were perfect matches. Too bad I didn't have any more brothers and sisters.

Derek offered to be tested to see if he was a match. "I appreciate the offer, but the chance that you'd be a match is one in twenty-five thousand. Ethnicity plays a role, and you're certainly not a Jew of Eastern European descent."

"I don't care, I want to get tested." He did and he wasn't a match.

I couldn't fathom dying from myelodysplasia just because no donor was found. Unfortunately, just like those individuals waiting for a new heart or liver, many expire. Just give me a chance.

My mom convinced me to visit one other transplant center before making a final decision, so Christine arranged a meeting with Dr. Bruce, a pediatric oncologist at NIH with a great knowledge of transplants. He

was prepared to give me his objective opinion of the best place for me. Dr. Bruce is another one of those jokesters—us Jews are known for our humor. When he saw my curly hair back in September 2000, he told me that he too had once had a He-Bro. He patiently answered my two pages of questions.

This was much different than the Ewing's sarcoma hospitalization when I let my parents decide everything. There were no repressed memories this time around. I wasn't submerging into the unknown world of cancer; I had showered in the shit for a year. I instructed my parents and Aunt Florence not to say anything until I was done speaking. They didn't fight me. They saw the focus in my eyes.

The cancer treatment utilized before the transplant is called the conditioning regimen. Most transplant centers employed the same or similar regimens. "If the regimen is the same, then what is the real difference between the transplant centers?" I asked.

"The chemo isn't the issue here. If I wanted to, I could give you chemo in my basement. I don't think that's legal, but that's another story. The real difference between these hospitals is experience of the doctors and nurses. The more transplants they have done, the better equipped they are to handle whatever problems you might have."

I went straight down my mom's list of transplant centers. Milwaukee specialized in T-cell depletion transplants, so I scratched that off. T-cells are a type of white blood cell. If I were to get a T-cell depleted transplant, then I would lose the graft vs. leukemia effect. That means if there was even a single cell that survived the conditioning regimen, then the new bone marrow would attack and kill it. If the T-cells were removed, then there would be nothing to find the diseased cells that might survive, and the transplant would be a waste. "In that sense, a little graft vs. host disease is good," Dr. Bruce said.

Graft vs. host disease, or GVHD, is one of the most severe complications of a transplant. The new marrow recognizes the person's body as

foreign, and attacks it. GVHD can be mild or severe. Half of the patients who receive an unrelated transplant develop GVHD, and ten to twenty percent of them die. Unfortunately, it's also difficult to diagnose. That's where hospital experience comes into play.

"GVHD is good?" I asked, surprised. "I thought it was really bad, like it could kill me."

"It can. GVHD is measured on a scale of stages from one to four.

Stage One GVHD is mild and consists only of a skin rash. You want to have some of this GVHD because it shows that your new marrow is active and working. If it's working properly, then you'll have a strong graft vs. leukemia effect. Stage Two is moderate—skin rash, liver and stomach problems. Stage Three is severe, and Stage Four is life-threatening."

Seattle performed the most transplants in the country. Seattle's traditional transplants were similar to Hopkins's, except Seattle used radiation and chemo for the conditioning regimen, whereas Hopkins only used chemo. Oddly, even though my previous chemo caused my second cancer, I was more afraid of total body irradiation. I dismissed Seattle.

The last transplant center was Minnesota. "Minnesota offers a different kind of transplant that's still fairly new. Their transplants use stem cells from umbilical cords instead of from the actual bone marrow. Once the umbilical cord is severed, its stem cells are frozen. When it's time for a transplant, the cells are thawed and given to the patient intravenously, in the same way he would receive a blood transfusion. If you're going to get a second opinion, which I strongly urge, I would visit the University of Minnesota, since they perform the most umbilical cord transplants."

"Okay, then. I've narrowed it down to Hopkins and Minnesota."

"Make sure you pack your sweater because it's going to be cold."

While taking a shower, I performed my occasional testicular examination. Right nut—good. Left nut—what the hell? My left testicle was at least five times larger than my right, resembling a lime. My response

was predictable—I had testicular cancer. So there you have it. I'm going to be one of the first people to survive three cancers before I could drink legally.

I wondered how it was possible to have two fucking cancers at the same fucking time. I thought of other possible reasons why my nut was enormous, and all I could come up with was Squashball.

During our senior year of high school, Drew and I invented a game called Squashball, where two, three or four people sit about twelve feet apart with their legs spread. The person in possession of the small, lightweight ball tosses it toward the groin of the player directly in front of him. That player is not allowed to move, catch or swat at the ball. If he gets hit, he has to take it like a man. The object of the game is to cause pain for the opposing player.

The night we invented Squashball, we had a blindfold round, in which the person receiving the toss had to close his eyes until the ball landed. Drew was pissed that I had already jacked him five times, so he decided to throw an illegal line drive. Without the ability to see this throw, I was unable to stop the ball, and it hit the target dead-on. Over the next few months of playing Squashball, my nuts endured significant punishment. Could Squashball cause inflated nuts? Could Squashball cause cancer?

I stopped thinking about it and tried to sleep. I was scheduled to be at NIH the following morning for blood counts, and I knew the outcome of my visit could change my life forever. If I had testicular cancer, then I would be having surgery to remove my enlarged testicle within days. I was able to take comfort in knowing that when testicular cancer is caught early, the prognosis is good.

I remembered what our rabbi said in one of his sermons. "Every night before you go to sleep, and every morning when you wake-up, say the Shema. When you say the prayer at night, ask God to take care of your loved ones. When you say it after you wake up, thank God that

you are alive and in good health for yet another day. The Shema is a declaration of faith; it's the first prayer Jews are taught to say and the last words said prior to death."

So that night, I decided to recite the Shema twice each day, although, I tend to forget about ninety-seven percent of my mornings.

שְׁמַע יִשְׂרָאֵל: יְיָ אֱלֹהֵינוּ יְיָ אֶחָד!

בָּרוּךְ שֵׁם כְּבוֹד מַלְכוּתוֹ לְעוֹלָם וָעֶד!

Hear O Israel: the Lord is our God, the Lord is One!
Blessed is His glorious kingdom for ever and ever!

After a restless night, I left the house eager to show Christine my big left nut. I had to know if it was cancer immediately. When I got to her office, I stood up, dropped my pants and stared at the wall.

A year earlier, I had gotten a massive erection during an exam. I still wonder if Christine had been trying to cause an erection by the way she had felt around for swollen lymph nodes. Times like that I wished my examiner was a fat, hairy Italian guy with garlic on his breath. But Christine was the opposite of that, so I tried to start thinking about football. When that didn't work, dinosaurs. Then…are you done yet? By that time, she had started checking my leg strength, rubbing my thigh for muscle size and tone. "Physical therapy is definitely getting you stronger," Christine had said. She had crept further up my thigh and by the time her hands got inside my boxers, I had felt movement. I could not tell if she had not noticed or if she had just thought I was tenting, but she had continued to massage me. She had really gotten into it, pushing with both hands on my upper quadriceps and hamstring. By now, I had gotten so nervous that I had begun to sweat. Just when I had reached an eighty-percent salute, Christine had announced that she was done. I had pulled up my jeans and left the room faster than I could say, "Oh shit, I have a boner."

There was no way I was going for a repeat performance this year. Christine turned the light off and grabbed a flashlight. "What are you doing?" I asked.

"I'm going to look through your testicle with a flashlight. Oftentimes you can tell if it's fluid."

She conducted her little experiment and sighed. "It looks like fluid, but I'm going to send you down for an ultrasound just to make sure."

I headed down to the radiology waiting room and signed my name on the list. Minutes later, a man who looked like he enjoyed working with jelly a bit too much called my name. I followed him to a dark room with an ultrasound machine and a table. "Lie on your back with your pants down."

He squirted gel onto the ultrasound probe and lightly pressed it on my nut sack. He moved the probe around my scrotum and abdomen. "What do you think it is?" I finally said.

"It looks like fluid."

"That's good. Fluid is good."

When the ultrasound was complete I went back up to Floor 13 and waited for Christine to give me the official results. "Okay, Ben. You don't have testicular cancer."

"Good news."

"I talked with the radiologist, and he says you have a hydrocele, which is an accumulation of fluid in your testicle. It was caused by inflammation of your epididymis. That's where your sperm is stored. It's not dangerous."

My Supersperm must be rebelling because I was not getting laid.

"Will it return to normal?"

"I imagine it will change size as the fluid enters and exits the epididymis."

My large testicle, although awkward, would cause me no harm. Kevin Garnett, clear the lane because I'm coming through.

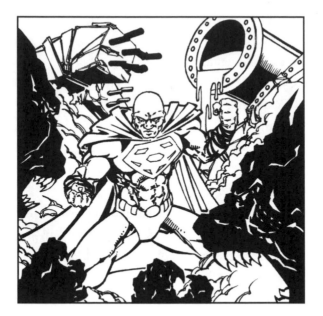

Chapter 7
LAND OF TEN-THOUSAND LAKES

During our flight to Minneapolis, I turned around to see how my
dad was doing. He was staring out the window with a curious look on
his face. "Benjy, let me show you something…look out the window and
at the wing. Do you see?"

"See what?"

"The wing is flapping around out there!"

Sure enough, the wing was slightly bouncing up and down. "It's supposed to do that," I said.

"No, I don't think so. That wing is flapping because it's going to fall off!"

I laughed too hard to even respond. As we approached Minneapolis-St.
Paul International Airport, I saw hundreds of frozen bodies of water, one
after another. The sky was gray and looked like it could start snowing at
any second. I knew that once I stepped out of the airport, I would feel

the cold, crisp air of the Midwest and watch as my breath formed a cloud, a pure sign of my existence.

After several mild winters, Virginia had been pounded by a blizzard in February that left us with eighteen inches of snow. That was when I first discovered there is something about those crystalline snowflakes dropping from the sky that makes me feel alive. Cancer had given me a new-found esteem for every season and condition, including heavy rain. "Who the hell likes rainy days?" Derek once asked me.

"I do. I like the smell of the rain. It smells peaceful."

The Minneapolis airport was monstrous. When we finally reached the exit and I walked through the automatic doors, my eyes watered with the temperature plunge. I took a deep breath and smiled because it felt good. Bracing.

Our hotel was on the University of Minnesota campus, two miles down the road from downtown Minneapolis. The city was spotless, with well-maintained streets, and litter-free sidewalks. There were as many cool stores and good restaurants as you would see in DC. I loved this city at first sight.

We had come to the pediatric transplant clinic to meet Dr. Fry, one of the most awesome doctors I had ever met. It didn't take him long to sell me on his transplant center. He was down-to-earth and soft-spoken. He told us all about umbilical cord blood transplants. In 1990, the University of Minnesota had performed the first cord blood transplant for leukemia. Its biggest advantage was the low incidence of GVHD. Even if the recipient developed GVHD, the severity would be less than that of a traditional transplant. There were proportionally fewer cases of Stage Three or Stage Four GVHD with cord transplants and many fewer deaths. It took less time to find a cord blood donor because the match didn't have to be as perfect—they can use 4/6 HLA matches while traditional transplants can't use anything less than a 5/6 HLA match.

The disadvantage of a cord transplant is that fewer stem cells are

collected from an umbilical cord than from an adult's pelvic bone. The fact that I was small was a good thing, because the bigger you are, the more stem cells you need.

"If cord blood transplants are so good, then why aren't they the next big thing in transplantation?" I asked.

"I think they are."

I told Dr. Fry about the thirty percent chance Dr. Connors from Hopkins had given me, and asked what he thought. He was reluctant to give a number, but I got it out of him. "It's about forty percent for full-blown leukemia and sixty percent for myelodysplasia for a patient who has not had previous chemo. Because of your previous cancer treatment I'd put you at fifty percent." At that mark I didn't even need Jonathan to help convince me I would survive. Half the patients live—it was clear as day I would be one of them.

Recovery would be similar to what Dr. Ford from Hopkins had described, although Dr. Fry didn't guarantee I would get depressed. I didn't ask about that, because I knew Dr. Fry would dismiss depression as nonsense. He was very optimistic. When I asked if I could return to UVA in the fall semester, he wanted to say yes, and then realized it would be impossible. I would have to stay in Minnesota for a minimum of fourteen weeks.

Dr. Fry stepped out of the room to allow me and my parents discuss everything. "What do you think?" I asked.

"Great!" my dad said.

"This place is wonderful!" my mom said. "I can tell they're going to take great care of you here."

The social worker came to talk to us. She said that she would be there to talk if I needed emotional support. "That's okay, I have got things under control," I said.

"I can tell. I'll still be there if you need me, but I won't ask you again."

"Thank you, I appreciate that."

The social worker had already placed my name on the cord blood donor registry. I was aware of the high cost of a transplant so when she showed me a listing of nearby apartments, I balked. NIH was government-funded, so the first round of cancer with the Ewing's sarcoma had not cost my parents much. Because my dad worked for the U.S. Department of Energy we had Federal BlueCross BlueShield health insurance, which paid ninety percent of expenses until we reached the out-of-pocket maximum of $4,000. After that, Federal BlueCross paid one hundred percent.

The University of Minnesota (and Hopkins for that matter) was a non-profit, private hospital, far from home, so my parents would incur travel and apartment expenses. I was worried about their financial well-being. "We don't need to stay in a nice apartment. I'm sure the Ronald McDonald House is suitable."

My mom, annoyed, said, "Benjamin, stop it." She turned to the social worker. "We will want an apartment."

My uncle offered to pay rent at the apartment. I told my dad not to accept it, but my uncle wouldn't budge. Then my mom's Jazzercise group and our Temple raised several hundred dollars for us. At the end, when we came back to Manassas, friends raised funds to have our house cleaned for our return. The last financial aid was difficult for me to accept but I was glad for anything that made my mom's life easier.

The social worker escorted us to the main hospital building through underground tunnels. From the hospital lobby we took the elevator to the fourth floor and proceeded to enter the pediatric transplant unit. It was as pleasant an environment as I have seen in a hospital. The layout was informal, with the nurses' desk in the middle. The wooden doors were a lively brown and the walls were blue, pink, or white. Ornaments dangled from the ceiling. On each door was a white board with the patient's name written in a unique way. Some of the doors had pictures of the patient, mostly from when he or she was healthy. I would be the

oldest patient on the pediatric unit by maybe five years, but I didn't mind. I was encouraged by the friendly atmosphere.

The social worker showed us the only unoccupied room. "This is pretty nice," I said. "Kind of small, but nice."

"This is the smallest room we have," she said. "Hopefully, you will get one of the larger ones."

"I have one question. I have this old and dirty stuffed animal that I got when I was four years old. It had been my dad's aunt's before she became ill. Am I allowed to keep it in the room with me?"

"Probably not. There are quite a few rules, like no plants, fruits, or anything that will grow bacteria or fungus. I suppose if you clean him really well you may be able to keep him in your room."

"No, that's okay. It's not a big deal."

I felt like a pussy for even asking. My stuffed monkey, George, used to go everywhere with me. When I had ear surgery at five years old, I brought George into the OR with me. When I woke up, George had a bandage wrapped around his head that was identical to the one around mine. He was so old there was no way to clean him. My mom tried once, but his arm nearly fell off. He's still sitting on my bookcase, collecting dust. Maybe George should wear my Super-Jew shirt.

Back home, after relinquishing my student ID, I had few responsibilities. I didn't have to think about midterms or plan for nighttime activities, because my friends were mostly away at college. I didn't have the pressure of hitting on girls and getting shot down. I just had to find ways to entertain myself and get blood counts and transfusions. I was actually at peace more than I had been at any other point in my life.

The transfusions kept my hemoglobin and platelets at manageable levels, and I had no other side effects. I didn't feel sick, tired or weak. I felt fantastic. I somewhat enjoyed my clinic visits, as I talked and joked with my doctors and nurses as if they were my buddies. I mostly ignored the

other patients, who, I imagined, were jealous of how normal I looked.

However, at three in the afternoon one day, I couldn't wait to leave NIH. Traffic was horrendous any Friday afternoon between Manassas and NIH, but it was worse this afternoon when it looked like a blizzard was coming. I was waiting patiently in the lobby, listening to 3 Doors Down, when my nurse tapped me on the shoulder and said, "Ben, your mom is on the phone."

I assumed she was going to tell me to drive carefully. "Hello."

"Hi sweetie, you're still there I guess."

"Yep."

"Is it snowing?"

"Yep."

"Oh, you better be careful coming home."

"Yep."

"Listen, I just got a call from Minnesota…they found a match and want to know whether you'd prefer to start in one week or two weeks."

"They already found a bone marrow match?"

"Isn't that great?" she said.

"Yeah, I guess. Already?"

"Dr. Fry wasn't lying when he said cord blood finds a match quicker."

"So, what do they want to know?"

"They have to set things up and need to know if you want to wait one week or wait two weeks before we fly there."

"No point in staying around here, anymore. I guess just a week."

I couldn't believe a match had already been found, and it made me kind of sad. That's not to say I didn't want to find a donor match and survive. I just didn't want my peaceful world to change, and I was scared. In one week I would fly halfway across the country and not return for months.

When Christine told me my blood counts were fine, I left NIH to embark on my long, slow trip back to Manassas. Formerly known as the site of the first major land battle of the Civil War, Manassas is now

recognized as the place where the D.C. Sniper killed a guy pumping gas and Lorena Bobbitt cut off her husband's penis in a fit of pique. Still, it was where my friends were and I would miss it during the long spring in Minneapolis. Even now, every time I hear 3 Doors Down, I can picture the window at the end of the NIH hallway with the snow hammering down in front of the dull gray sky as I headed home. The next day I sent an e-mail to my friends:

> Date: Saturday, March 29, 2003
> To: 26 of my friends
> I have a disease called myelodysplasia and the only cure is a bone marrow transplant. They found a donor match and I'm going to be treated at the University of Minnesota. I won't be back until August. As long as the old liver holds up, we will all drink excessive amounts of alcohol on that day. I'll still have my phone and e-mail there so holler at me from time to time. Spread the word to anyone else who would want to know.

Terry threw a small going-away party for me. She planned it on her own. I had developed a good friendship with Terry at UVA. She was the only girl I was comfortable around, which mostly has to do with her dating Nick and my forced proximity to her. Her courage in sticking it out with someone with AIDS is amazing.

Some of my friends showed up to her house that night, including several from UVA, one who drove all the way from Virginia Tech just for the party, and even the lovely Lily. I felt much love for those who came but many people I expected didn't show up, including some of my closest friends. One didn't come because he had a fraternity event; I later asked another friend what prevented him from attending and he said, "I can't remember." Another guy told me that the trip to DC for the party was "just too far." It didn't bother me at the time, as my hurt feelings were hidden behind my cape.

All my life, I had been picked on by other kids. I endured slurs about

being short and jokes about being Jewish, and I usually didn't mind. I know I'm short, and if I hear a clever Jew joke, I'll laugh too. During my senior year, though, the hostility from my core group of friends grew exponentially, possibly because they wanted to make up for being so nice to me when I had cancer.

I reached a point where I no longer enjoyed being around Andy, Drew and Worm. It was my loyalty to them—some of the same people I have known almost my whole life—that kept me from leaving the group. I could have left them at any time and become an equal member of Birdsall's group.

After years of their second class treatment of me, not showing up to Terry's party for me was the most fucked-up thing they had ever done. In their defense, they didn't know the significance of a bone marrow transplant. I made a point of not telling them how dangerous it was in my e-mail. Several months after returning home from Minnesota, I was at Andy's house watching football, and we got on the subject of my transplant. When I told him there had been a coin-flip chance he'd ever see me again, he replied, "I had no idea your odds were that slim." If they had known I was given a fifty percent chance of dying, then maybe they'd have come running.

My dad began his lonely two-day drive to Minneapolis in The Big Red Box which was packed to the brim. Derek, Birdsall and Bently came to my house to watch the Final Four games, including Texas vs. Syracuse. That year, Jonathan organized a Final Four Tournament pool with over forty participants. I had Texas winning in my bracket and had to watch $400, as well as bragging rights for life, go up in flames as they lost to Syracuse 95-84. Derek was reluctant to leave when the games were over. Maybe he understood what a fifty percent chance meant more than I did.

Two days later, I left my house for a four-month journey of a lifetime. Unlike my first bout with cancer, this time I acknowledged the possibility that I might not make it. I nearly threw out my collection of

Sports Illustrated swimsuit issues hidden in my drawer. Just in case I died, I didn't want my parents finding them. I decided to take the gamble.

At dawn, my dad's friend from Temple drove me and my mom to the airport. I closed the door to his gold Cadillac and looked out the tinted window. The sun had just begun to rise, and I couldn't quite make out the four tall, white pillars on the front porch, or the two pink dogwoods in the yard, or through the window of my bedroom where George was sitting on the bookshelf. Bye, House.

My dad had arrived in Minneapolis with the Big Red Box the night before, so he picked us up at the airport. We ate breakfast at McDonald's on the way to the clinic for my first day of intense testing. I wasn't hungry and barely ate my hotcakes. How could I be hungry? In two weeks, I was going to be fucked up beyond a masochist's wildest fantasies.

A few days later, we went to Ground Round for dinner and the waitress asked what we were doing in Minneapolis. "Benjamin is getting a bone marrow transplant at the University of Minnesota," my mom said, jabbering about my health issues to total strangers just like she always did. The waitress took a seat on the booth, wrapped her arm around me and sincerely wished me luck. Yeah, the Midwest was different from the East.

It took me one minute to acclimate to the time change, but my dad claims that he never did get fully adjusted. For the entire four months in Minnesota, he refused to turn his watch back one hour. I recalled that on our ten-day Israel trip, he left his watch on Eastern Standard Time, even though there was a seven-hour difference.

The first test performed at the clinic was a blood draw, more fittingly described as a blood drain, considering there was a basketful of vials. It felt like the needle punctured my bicep. I was forced to watch a video on bone marrow transplantation before signing my seven-page consent form, which contained the word "fatal" six times. Two other patients watched the video with me, both old men with one foot in the

grave. Watching the video, and being in the presence of Future Fatalities of America, was a shock to my already sinking confidence. This was no Hell Week. I was entering Hell Months.

I read several disturbing things in the consent form: (1) Taking part in any clinical research involves risks and may provide some benefits; (2) It could turn out that the changes made are not good ones, and that they actually could end up making the transplant less effective or less safe in some way; (3) The umbilical cord blood (the "graft") may fail to grow up inside your body at all; (4) If graft failure occurs, this will result in low blood counts for a long period of time and can be fatal; (5) It is possible that certain genetic diseases may be passed through the transplanted umbilical cord blood stem cells; (6) Each umbilical cord blood can only be tested for a few of the many possible genetic diseases; (7) Though rare, it is possible that incorrect labeling of an umbilical cord blood unit could occur; (8) This could result in malfunction of any organ in your body such as heart, lungs, liver, gut, kidneys and bladder, brain etc.; (9) Your disease may recur even if initially your transplant is successful.

The form should have been titled, "Transplants: Everything Imaginable Except a Dick in Your Ass." I could list the thirty-three different side effects of the drugs and treatment, but I don't think that will be necessary. Our apartment building was designated university housing, but six spaces were allotted to transplant patients. It was two blocks away from the medical center and far more charming than The Hump. It was fully furnished and even had a La-Z-Boy. Sitting on my La-Z-Boy…just like old times. Our first visitor stopped by while we were unpacking. He was a chunky Asian who looked to be about my age. "Hi, I live right next door."

"It's nice to meet you," my dad said. "That's Ben over there; he's here for a bone marrow transplant."

"Hey," I said.

"That's what I figured," the chunky guy said.

"Where are you from?" my dad asked.

"I'm from Okinawa. My sister is here with me."

"Is that right? So have you already received a bone marrow transplant?

"Yes, I got mine about six months ago."

"Six months? I thought you get to leave after a hundred days," my dad said.

"Some people do, but I had many complications. They say I may be able to leave in two or three months. I developed GVHD, and the medication they put me on had all kinds of side effects. I'm on three meds now just to control my blood pressure. Take a look at my calves."

His lower legs looked like tree trunks. "The medication did that?" my dad asked.

"Yes. My calves blew up from all these drugs. I hope Ben doesn't need to take this stuff. Anyway, hopefully I'll see you all around."

Once my dad closed the door, he said, "He seems like a nice boy."

"It might be nice having a friend next door," my mom said.

I never wanted to see that guy again. He looked like the spokesperson for shitty transplants, and hearing him talk about it was depressing. I didn't want GVHD. I didn't want to stay one second past the hundred days. And I didn't want the fattest calves on the planet, either.

When my parents and I ate at Perkins that night, I became intensely fearful of the transplant. With each passing day, my highly toxic conditioning regimen drew nearer. I ordered chicken parmesan, but ate less than half of it. I learned everything I could going into the transplant, but it still seemed like a mystery to me. With a bone marrow transplant on the horizon, a new home halfway across the country where the unusually amiable natives speak with an odd accent, where my closest friend is a thousand miles away, I was one scared, sad kid. I couldn't wait for Jonathan to come visit later in the week but my mom was set on convincing him not to fly to Minneapolis. "There's no reason for you to visit now. You have school. Once you graduate, you can be with Benjamin for

the rest of our stay here." I didn't try to stop her but secretly I wanted Jonathan to see me while I was still healthy, even if he could only stay for a few days.

When we got back to the apartment, I watched Syracuse beat Kansas 81-78 in the national championship basketball game. I was rooting for Syracuse because my dad went there for graduate school, even though they eliminated Texas in the Final Four, preventing me from winning Jonathan's pool. Kansas had a chance for a three-pointer to win the game when Syracuse's Hakim Warrick came out of nowhere to block the shot.

My dad went with me the next day to the OR for my bone marrow biopsy and spinal tap, which were performed just to be certain that I still had zero leukemic cells. I was glad that I was given general anesthesia. Extracting juice from my spine didn't seem pleasurable. My biopsy showed an almost-empty marrow, but there were no leukemic cells and I was still on track to receive my transplant in exactly two weeks.

My ANC had dropped under five hundred. I was neutropenic. Just three months after being red-flagged for low platelets, my rapid cancer had already destroyed nearly every hematopoietic stem cell in my body. It was difficult to accept that my bone marrow, the core of my Super Man complex, was self-destructing. Platelets were wiped out. Red cells were wiped out. Now, white cells were gone. "Complain all you want," I told this cancer of mine. "In two weeks you'll be dead, Myelodysplasia."

Jonathan wanted to see me one last time before my transplant. He brought most of his DVDs with him—nearly a hundred. We both knew that movies would be my main source of entertainment.

"This location is amazing," Jonathan said.

"I know. There are so many restaurants within walking distance."

Our apartment was in fast food heaven, and I planned on taking full advantage. I was cautioned that I might not be able to eat. Dr. Fry informed me that most patients go on TPN.

"What's TPN?" I had asked.

"Total Parenteral Nutrition," Dr. Fry had said. "It's an IV bag that contains everything you need to survive and maintain weight—fat, protein, vitamins, minerals, sugar, everything. We have some patients who stay on TPN for a few months."

"I don't think I'll need it. For my last cancer, I was able to maintain my weight throughout all fourteen cycles."

"I just want to give you a heads-up. It's possible that you'll also need pain medicine for your mouth sores. Nearly all our patients stay on some form of morphine until their mouth sores go away."

"Really? I had some nasty mouth sores in the past, but I rarely needed pain medicine for them." Been there, done that.

Jonathan joined us at the clinic, and another future transplantee plunked down next to him. An eight-year-old from Georgia, he seemed determined to tell Jonathan the story of his short life in twenty minutes. He talked so quickly I was not even sure he was breathing. Every once in a while Jonathan would say, "Yeah," or "Mm-hmm," just to show he was still conscious. There was something refreshingly innocent about this kid. He just didn't comprehend that he might not ever get back home to his ATV.

On the other hand, I did comprehend that my chances of survival were limited and then I had to convince myself that they did not apply to me. I was getting a transplant because I didn't want to die. I doubt that death ever crossed this kid's mind. To him, the transplant was simply a temporary halt to driving around in his ATV. It was what Lance Armstrong says: children cope with cancer better than adults because all they want to do is finish treatment so they can go out and play.

As part of my conditioning regimen, I would receive total body irradiation. My parents and I met with the radiation oncology specialist to discuss it. Instead of beams shooting at me from different angles like for Ewing's sarcoma, this radiation would blanket my entire body. No escape. I would absorb 1,350 rads over four days, with two sessions each

day, which sounded more like Adrian Peterson's routine at the NFL Combine.

The technician manufactured a lead block so that my lungs only sustained partial radiation. It was possible I would require an inhaler for the rest of my life. Another possible late effect could be a forty percent chance of developing cataracts within five years.

"What area of your body did you receive radiation before?" the radiation oncology specialist asked.

"My left hip and part of my bowel."

"Have you had any X-rays of your hip lately?"

"Every time I see my surgeon. He said that what's left of my hip is necrotic."

"Organs have a radiation tolerance. If they receive more radiation than they can endure, then they start to fail. The bowel has been known to tolerate 5,500 rads."

"But I'll get more than that. I'm getting 4,500 plus 1,350. That's...by my calculations...5,850 rads! What will happen to my bowel?"

"Probably nothing, but there's a twenty-five percent chance that a portion of your bowel will stop working. In that case, you will need surgery to repair it."

"Is that it?"

"There's another twenty-five percent chance that the surgery wouldn't save your bowel and so you would need a colostomy bag."

"What's a colostomy bag?"

"A sack you wear on your hip that collects your excrement. Most people can live normal and productive lives with a colostomy bag."

"You mean that I wouldn't be able to shit on my own?"

"That's correct."

"No! No way! I'd rather kill myself than walk around with a shit bag forever," I said as the rage, red as blood, infested my head.

"Benjamin, don't you say that!" my mom said.

"It's true, I'm dead serious. There is no way that I would do that."

"There is one more thing we can do," the specialist said. "We can create a lead block to cover the part of your hip and bowel that was radiated. That way, no radiation will pass through."

"What about killing the myelodysplatic cells?" I asked.

"None of those cells are living in your bowel because there's no marrow. And, like you said, your bone is already dead from your previous radiation."

"Okay, let's do that."

The specialist called Dr. Fry to make sure that he approved of the lead block. After he concurred, she contacted NIH for my radiation records faxed over, and ordered a CT scan for my hip, just to make sure the bone was dead. When the scan was finished, I asked the radiation technician, "Did the bone look dead?"

"You have almost no bone there to begin with. And what's left absolutely looked dead. "

This was the most critical decision of my life and I was fifty-one percent certain I made the right one. Even if somehow there were myelo-dysplastic cells living in my bowel or dead bone, the chemo would hopefully wipe them out. This was the only time I refused to follow through with the preferred, cautious treatment. The consequences of the decision to receive less radiation than the docs advised could have been fatal.

There's always uncertainty when dealing with cancer therapy. As a patient you are offered the traditional, doctor-recommended approach accompanied by horrible side effects and countless unforeseeable late effects. Then there's the experimental, less-rigorous, or unproven approach in which the side effects will be less severe, if you live to see them. If I had refused to get all fourteen cycles of chemo for Ewing's sarcoma, for instance, then maybe I wouldn't have developed myelodys-plasia. Then again, maybe I would be dead.

Some people think traditional treatment is overkill and have no problem trying alternative methods. In my opinion, the risks of not

taking the traditional approach are almost never worth it. I just hoped my one act of rebellion wouldn't turn out to be a mortal mistake.

My dad went with me for the insertion of my Hickman catheter. We waited in the OR where the television was always on CNN, as if to show you that getting cut up was nothing compared to the latest breaking news. It was getting to the point where surgery was standard for me; I didn't need CNN to gain perspective.

A Hickman is much like a port—the tube is tunneled through the vein beneath the collarbone and ends at the heart. The difference is that the Hickman catheter protrudes out of the skin through a small surgical incision, and then separates into two different IV lines, allowing two drugs to infuse simultaneously.

My Hickman disgusted me. I would have much preferred to have a port, but because of the need for a constant IV, often two at once, I didn't have a choice. For four months, I refused to look at the plastic tube jabbed through my chest while my new skin cells were slowly growing around it. My nurses always said to me, "Your Hickman looks great. Do you want to see?"

"No thanks."

I woke up after surgery in my new home—Room 210 on the fourth floor at University of Minnesota Medical Center. The room was much larger than the one I had seen during my first Minnesota visit. I could hear rumbling from the vent in the ceiling, called a HEPA filter, which kept my room germ-free. It beat being in a plastic bubble. An enormous window provided a picturesque view of the Mississippi River, no more than a hundred yards away.

A nursing assistant came in to welcome me. "What does a nursing assistant do?" I asked.

"Oh, the usual. Measure your poop and pee and take your temperature and blood pressure," she said.

"What do you mean measure my poop? I have to go in that plastic

container?"

"You'll get used to it."

"Every single time?"

"Yep."

"Gross. And you don't mind cleaning it up?"

"Nope. You can call me the poop and pee girl!"

We went out to dinner that evening, but once I arrived back at the hospital , I was not allowed to leave for any reason, except to go down to the first floor for radiation or scans. We ate at Leaning Tower of Pizza. I couldn't bring myself to order their specialty celery pizza, and settled on pepperoni. Before heading back, I took a shit in my apartment. I wanted to hold off on depositing into the plastic container for as long as possible.

My parents took me back to my room, helped me get settled, and then left. At NIH, my parents were in my room all the time. Here, I laid down rules for all visitors, including family members. No arguing, yelling or nagging. Nothing that raises my stress level. Answer the phone so I don't have to. Don't put me in a situation where I'm forced to talk on the phone. No eating in the room without my permission because other people's food made me nauseous. Leave before I go to bed, and arrive after I wake up. My parents had trouble with the last one.

I was cozy in my new single-bedroom home. I believe my room was possibly the best on the transplant unit. I had an adjustable bed, a large chair with a footrest, a treadmill, computer, and TV. I had my PS2 and an assortment of DVDs, and I had pretty girls watching over me from their desk just outside of my door.

I watched *Training Day* before going to sleep. That night it was easy to forget that I would soon be getting inhumane doses of chemo and radiation. For the moment, I was in heaven.

The three days of chemo and four days of radiation would completely eliminate my bone marrow. I'm not talking about that piece-of-cake neutropenia. I'm talking about destroying every white cell, red

cell and platelet. The conditioning regimen would create a ticking time bomb with no known time of detonation. For the next three weeks, my germ-free room and countless blood and platelet transfusions would be the only things to stall the explosion. I would undoubtedly die if the transplant hadn't come along to save me. I couldn't believe I was getting chemo again just eighteen months after Cycle Fourteen's final bag of etoposide was tossed into the biohazard receptacle.

I caught a break, when fludarabine was the only chemo on the menu. With the exception of Zofran, which I would receive continuously for the next eight days, I didn't need any anti-nausea medicine. Fludarabine was mild. Lying on a bed, getting some chemo...just like old times. But I went to sleep scared shitless. Over the next two days I would be getting Cytoxan, which is not mild, along with fludarabine. Cytoxan is pure poison.

The nurse had given me a half-dose of Phernergan, an anti-nausea drug, promising me it wouldn't knock me out. It kept me practically comatose for the next six hours. I couldn't open my eyelids, no matter how hard I tried. I woke with an extreme urge to pee. "I have to pee," I said.

"Okay, we'll leave," replied my mom.

Without standing up, I grabbed the urinal directly next to me, got it in position and started pissing. Just like old times. I'm glad my urinal skills picked up where they left off. I didn't need to tilt my body for better positioning or even look to make sure the urinal wasn't overflowing. Through a combination of factors, including the warmth of the container, the amount of urine and the relative humidity of the air, I knew what I was doing.

"Is chemo finished?" I asked when I woke up.

"All done," my mom replied. "How do you feel?"

"Okay."

Actually, I felt like a Clydesdale had had his way with me. It was the same putrid feeling I remembered having in my last go around: the same desire to do nothing, the same sickness in my stomach, the same dizzy

sensation, the same yearning for time to fly by, the same stench that sweated through my skin and smothered my sheets.

My mom left around dinnertime. "I'll be back later," she said. I didn't care if she came back or not. I didn't want to talk to anyone.

Some of my nurses were gorgeous. I can think of seven who were very attractive, one of whom was in a class by herself: Jen Albright. Jen looked like Jessica Biel-turned-surfer-chick with her tan complexion, shoulder-length brown hair, and casual, laid-back quality. I always got nervous around Jen because she was so gorgeous. I maintained a crush on her for the next two years. If I were given another crack at it now, I know I would act cooler. Years of female scorn have trained me. A couple shots of Captain Morgan wouldn't hurt, either.

But on this day, appearance meant nothing, and I hated Jen for one reason—she made me take a shower. The hospital rule was I had to shower every other day. Feeling terrible and standing in a frigid bathroom made it a miserable experience. I shivered my way through it.

I knew things that would lead you to believe I was stalking her, like she wore only plain green or blue scrubs, and she always ordered takeout. I don't know if I was more jealous of Jen for being able to eat tasty food, or the food for being in Jen's mouth. Too bad she had to measure my vomit, piss, and shit on a daily basis. My mom rejoined me after dinner, so I sent my dad to get me a strawberry sundae from McDonald's. Just like old times. Within thirty minutes of eating the ice cream, I became nauseous.

After forty-five minutes of controlled breathing to stave off the sickness, I had everyone leave the room so that I could gag myself. I noticed the dark red liquid of the strawberry sundae floating on the chunky surface of the bucket but when Jen measured the pH, she concluded that it was blood. This wasn't just like old times. This was way worse.

I tried to sleep. It might have been easier if my mom had stuck around but I clung to my principle of going to sleep by myself. I was so frightened that I nearly called to ask if she would come back. For the

Ewing's sarcoma, all I had wanted was to get rid of her, but now that she wasn't there, I wanted her.

When the chemo was complete, I felt grateful that it only had lasted for three days rather than ten months. I was already feeling its effects, one being my failing taste buds. My mom bought me three different beverages before I could finally taste one, which was Mountain Dew. My saliva no longer resembled a liquid; it stuck to my puke buckets like caulk. I wouldn't have been surprised if it hardened.

Cytoxan was most acutely toxic to my bladder. I was supposed to pee at least three hundred milliliters every two hours, which wasn't easy because Cytoxan also caused edema. By the afternoon, I hadn't reached that mark, so Jen gave me Lasix, a diuretic. I needed two more doses of Lasix later in the day.

Late in the afternoon, I defecated. What exited my body was a substance I didn't know humans could produce. "I just shit brown water," I said as I left the bathroom.

"Is that normal?" my dad asked.

"I don't know."

I buzzed Jen. "I just went to the bathroom and it was brown liquid. Like straight water. Have you seen that before?"

"Yeah, that happens to everyone."

I was relieved that I had diarrhea and not constipation. Heading into the transplant, one of my biggest fears was that I would get constipated and tear my rectum. Without an immune system for several weeks, my anus would have no chance of healing.

With the exception of some Mountain Dew, I ate and drank nothing. I looked at my stack of Deer Park water bottles in the corner and realized they weren't going anywhere. In fact, I wondered when Dr. Fry was going to start me on TPN. I had already lost five pounds since arriving in Minnesota. If I had been the size of William "The Refrigerator" Perry, then I would have nothing to worry about. The depression that the

doctors at Hopkins had mentioned couldn't possibly begin this soon, I reasoned, because I lacked the energy to feel anything.

The next morning, another nasty surprise. I crapped blood. I screamed. "What's the matter?" Jen came running.

"I just went to the bathroom, and it's dark red. I think it's blood."

"Okay. Let me see."

I bit my lip. "What have you eaten today?" she asked.

"I had red Jell-O a couple hours ago. That's all I've eaten today."

"That's the culprit right there. This isn't blood." The Jell-O had gone straight through me. I should try blue Kool-Aid next time, just for fun.

During and after my conditioning regimen, I was averaging six diarrhea shits a day that resembled a low viscosity liquid. Mostly I pooped during the day, but sometimes I would wake up at night with the extreme urge. I could count the number of seconds I had to reach the toilet on both hands. During the day one of my parents would quickly unplug my IV pump and I would rush to the bathroom. But at night I was alone, I was groggy, and I wasn't given any notice. This was an abominable combination.

One night, I woke up with the creature knocking on my asshole like the FBI on John Gotti's front door. At first I fought it, clenching my anus as hard as I could. I needed to get off the bed, bend down to unplug the power cord, and walk ten feet to the bathroom, all without compromising my watertight rectum. The mission was doomed from the start.

Leaking isn't a strong enough word for what happened next. I would describe it as pressurized shots of liquid shit. The first one seeped through my boxers and onto the bed sheet. Then it started running down my leg, leaving a trail all the way to the toilet. When I finished pooping I cleaned the floor and threw out my boxers. I didn't want to tell Jen I shit myself, so I slept on the top sheet. In the morning when my nursing assistant changed my sheets, I pretended to be occupied with important e-mails.

That wasn't the only time that happened. The second time I didn't

clench nearly hard enough, and my asshole was far from watertight. Right as my feet touched the floor, I erupted like a volcano. The shit accumulated on the floor in what looked like a small mud puddle.

I buzzed the front desk. "Can you send my nurse in?"

I paced around my hospital room trying to figure out what to say. When she arrived, she looked down at the puddle, then at me. "I couldn't hold it."

Before changing the sheet, she called in the janitor. My immune system was fucked-up, so I couldn't leave the room. I had to watch as he mopped my shit. I couldn't even look him in the eye.

After a much-needed respite from treatment on the Sabbath, my nurse woke me up. "Time for radiation. There's a man here to escort you." I dressed and grabbed my particulate mask. I wasn't about to take one step outside my room without my germ-preventing mask secured tightly around my face. When I opened my door, I saw the man waiting for me with a wheelchair.

"I'll walk."

We went down to Radiation Oncology, where I was about to receive my first of eight radiation sessions. I went to the back room, and it was just as I imagined: lots of empty space, a huge machine, and a door that was built to guard Fort Knox.

There was a wooden platform I had to stand on, with side panels and pegs that ran up them. Once I stood on top, the technician secured the lead block for my lungs. "What about the block for my hip?" I asked her.

"That's not finished yet, but we'll have it done by this afternoon. Once you're in the correct position, you absolutely cannot move. If you do, then the block won't be in front of your lungs. I'm going to put a large screen in front of you which will scatter the rays."

"Does it matter if I close my eyes?"

"No. The radiation is going through your whole body, no matter what you do." For five minutes, I had to stand with my arms slightly out

to the side, completely motionless. After a brief break, I turned around for five more minutes.

"Have you had a patient not make it through all ten minutes?"

"I know it's tough, but you'll do it."

The technician exited the room and secured the door. I stood face-to-face with the machine. I felt it turn on—my hairs stood on end and a wave of nausea burst through my stomach. I wanted to close my eyes, but then again, what was the point? Instead I stared into the big, black eye of the machine from two feet behind the screen that scattered the beam, presumably for dose uniformity. I stood in the exact same position for five consecutive minutes, counting down the seconds in my mind.

The slightest movement would give my lungs too much radiation, and other parts of my chest cavity not enough. This, followed by another five minutes facing the wall behind me, was one of the most difficult tasks of my life. I was nauseous and weak from the chemo. I hadn't eaten anything for three days and had been puking to exhaustion. All I wanted to do was lie on my bed in my sterile room with the wonderful view.

When the second set of five minutes was complete, the technician sent me back upstairs. "Do you want me to get a wheelchair for you?" she asked.

"No thanks, I'll walk." She would have to knock me unconscious to get me into that wheelchair. Crank up the *Rocky* music.

In the early afternoon, I started playing video games, but got nauseous soon after. I blamed it on the extra concentration involved with playing PS2, and thus made a No Video Games rule. I wondered how many other prohibitive rules I could create for myself.

Thirty minutes later, I puked again. Never, in all of my cancer experience, had I vomited twice in such quick succession. "Add another tally mark to the Puke Count," I told my dad.

I kept a running count of my vomits on the white board in my room, which started as a joke. Jen found it hysterical. Around fifteen vomits, it stopped being funny. When it stopped six months later at ninety-three,

we were back to laughing again.

The radiation oncology specialist was waiting for me when I went down for my second radiation session in the afternoon. She finished the lead block for my hip, but also offered a different option in which she'd cut it in half, allowing only 300 to 400 rads of radiation to pass. "This is the amount we use for patients who have already received a lifetime of cancer treatment and can't handle much more. We call them mini-transplants, and survival rates are similar. If you did have any living cancer cells in your hip, this partial block would allow enough radiation to kill them." It was a perfect solution: not enough radiation to render a colostomy bag necessary, but just enough to kill cancer cells.

Two days later, the attending physician entered my room with a favor to ask. "Do you watch the show, *The Bachelor*?"

"No. Why?"

"Andrew Firestone, the guy in the show, is at this hospital today visiting different patients. He's considering giving the hospital a large donation. Would it be all right if I brought him in here to talk to you?"

"That's fine. Will he mind that I don't know who he is?"

"No, he's very nice."

Apparently, Mr. Firestone—The Bachelor and great-grandson of the founder of Firestone Tire and Rubber Company—was a big deal. Many of the nurses were beaming with joy in anticipation of his arrival. Even my mom had seen a couple episodes of *The Bachelor* and said that he seemed like a nice, handsome young man. I felt too awful to give a shit.

Andrew Firestone was in fact very nice. Before leaving, he gave my mom his e-mail address. "Let me know when Ben gets out, I'd love to send him a bottle of wine from my vineyard." Mom sent him an e-mail when I got out. "Ben is home and doing well," He never replied.

Hey tire man—I'm still waiting for your booze.

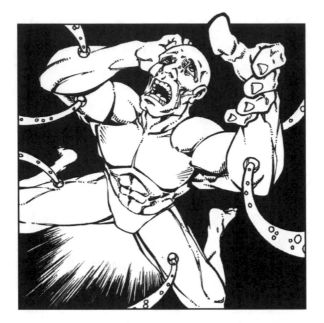

Chapter 8
TRANSPLANT DAY

The hospital presented every patient with a Transplant Day gift, and mine was a football that the Vikings played with in a regular season game. Since the ball was dirty, it was wrapped in two Ziploc bags and had to be taken out of the room immediately. It now sits in a trophy case on my dresser at home in front of my Wall of Fame. My social worker gave me a plush chicken, her kind way of making up for George not being allowed to stay with me. I named him Fatty the Chicken, and called him Fat Ass for short.

In late morning, Jen brought in a pathetically small bag of red liquid with a large O+ sticker on the front. Six months later my blood type would change from A+ to O+, that of my donor. I did a double take. This little thing is supposed to save my life? My unrelated umbilical cord

was a 4/6 HLA match from an infant girl born in New York in 1999. That was all I knew of her. With God on my side, I was ready for that baby girl to rescue me.

Before Jen released the valve to allow the stem cells to flow through my veins, she asked, "Is there anything you would like to say first?"

I longed to say the Shema, but instead said, "Do your job, little fella." My No Complaining rule prohibited me from making a big deal out of it. It was no joke, and I knew that. Jen released the valve and the stem cells swarmed into my Hickman.

Back when I had Ewing's sarcoma, every time I traveled to NIH, I brought my portable CD player, headphones and CD case. I worried that at some point I would become so despondent I would have trouble bouncing back. In case that happened, I left "*The Rocky Story,*" which contains the music from *Rocky* through *Rocky IV,* in my CD case at all times. Rocky was the easiest character to root for in all the movies I have ever seen. The character and music have always inspired me.

In the ninth grade, I had tutored a girl for her Bat Mitzvah. I had decided she was too soft-spoken and needed to speak louder, so I blasted the soundtrack, "*The Rocky Story,*" to get her excited for the big day. She thought I was out of my mind. When she told me she had no idea where the music came from, or who Rocky was, I thought she was the one who was out of her mind.

For sustained attitude, Superman was my role model. But for fighting for the title, getting through the worst moment, Rocky was my inspiration. I had gotten a little down a few months after my hip surgery and the mere memory of Rocky had brought me right back. With Rocky inspiring me, I transformed my sadness into anger, and my anger to energy. For some people, anger can be a negative emotion, but for me it was motivating. Sadness felt like defeat but my anger, when I turned it toward cancer, liberated me from being a Sick Kid and exposed me as a Super Man. Other cancer patients asked God

"Why?" I laughed at them for their weakness. I told cancer to go to hell. At UVA I hung a poster above my bed of Stallone standing on the front steps of the Philadelphia Museum of Art with his hands raised. Once when Derek and I were watching TV, a hallmate stopped and read the top line of the poster aloud. "'His whole life was a million-to-one shot.' You can't have Rocky hanging on your wall," he said. "You have nothing in common with him."

"Is that so? Well, the only thing you have in common with him is you're both from Philly," I countered.

"Damn right, we're both from Philly."

"I guess you're right. I'll take the poster down immediately."

When he left, I looked over at Derek and started laughing. "If he only knew." The Rocky poster stayed on my wall.

On Transplant Day, I needed Rocky. I stared at the poster, the only decoration in my room. And, while the little girl's stem cells flooded my body, I listened to my *Rocky* CD. I closed my eyes and drifted into a fantasy. My strong heart pumped my future marrow through my bloodstream. The cells targeted my hip, sternum and skull. They latched on like spiders, and began to repopulate my empty calcium-phosphorus shells. It was glorious. My fantasies of my nurses taking off their clothes for me had not panned out, but I sure hoped this one would.

Now, there was only one thing left to do—pray that this girl, whom I would never meet and whose name I'll never know, had the right kind of cells to give me a third chance at life.

There was undoubtedly something special in the way my body had reacted to Ewing's sarcoma, its treatment and its aftermath. My semen sample was larger than normal with a higher concentration of sperm. My white blood cells dropped to a dangerously low level after only half of the fourteen cycles. The other patients dropped for every one of the fourteen cycles.

My bone marrow recovery was extremely rapid. When I was admitted

for neutropenia, I was only in the hospital for a few days. The other patients stayed for a week. I needed fewer blood and platelet transfusions than many other patients. The chemo killed my cancer on impact. Some people's cancers never respond, and they die. I rehabilitated my hip at a record pace. My body adapted to surgery better than even my surgeon thought was possible. I never suffered from depression for any longer than a week. In fact, ongoing depression affects up to a quarter of cancer patients.

These extraordinary events occurred so frequently that I had to believe God had given me special powers. My emotional stability, the idea that I was above complaining and other normal invalid behaviors was noted by people who knew me and professionals too. My famous surgeon bragged about me. The praise of others fueled my feeling of superiority. Just as Lance Armstrong was once the best athlete in the world, I considered myself the Greatest Cancer Patient Ever. From the signs I was given, I didn't see any other way to perceive it. I was a Super Man.

By the time total body irradiation began, my white blood cell count had been three hundred and my doctors had decided to stop checking. They knew it would drop all the way down to zero, and determining the exact day that happened didn't justify taking extra blood. They would start checking again in a few days.

I talked with Jen when the next blood test came up. She told me to expect a white blood cell count of around 200. I thought it would be higher than that. The few mouth sores I had developed had already started going away, and when I was at NIH, mouth sores had not gone away until my white blood cells reached 1,000.

"Even white counts of 200 can take care of mouth sores," Jen said.

I didn't believe her. If a white cell count of 200 hadn't healed them in the past, why would they now? "What happens if my white count is more than 200?" I asked.

"Well if it's significantly higher, like over 1,000, then it's possible that

your old bone marrow wasn't entirely wiped out."

"You mean the myelodysplastic cells may still be alive?"

"It's possible, but very unlikely. Sometimes all the white cells recognize where your body is damaged and run to that spot to repair it. Okay?"

"Yeah."

"Seriously, don't worry about it."

In my heart, I already knew that my white blood cell count was much higher than 200, maybe closer to 1,000. It was the only logical explanation. After our conversation, I considered that my myelodysplasia had come back. I equally considered that my super powers injected themselves into my new bone marrow, causing a massive increase in white blood cell production. If my body had been superior during Ewing's sarcoma, why wouldn't it be superior now?

I couldn't get my brain out of overdrive. If I had myelodysplasia, who was going to tell me? How would he present it? What would I do? Could I handle a mini-transplant? Could my body tolerate more radiation? Would it be my fault because I pressured the radiation oncologist to create a lead block for my hip? What if Jen was right, and I only had a white count of 200? Did that mean I was just a regular patient? That my super powers had been killed along with the cancer cells?

A new nurse came in following the shift change to take my temperature. She looked nearly identical to Stacy Keibler, the WWE wrestler, Baltimore Ravens cheerleader and *Dancing with the Stars* contestant. I stared at her for a minute, unable to speak. "Can't sleep, huh?" she asked.

"No."

"Jen told me you were concerned about tomorrow's blood test." I nodded.

"You don't need to worry so much; I've seen mouth sores disappear when the patient has a white count of only a hundred. It's not that uncommon."

As she walked out the door, she looked over her shoulder and said

"I'm Trish, by the way." Her assurance relaxed me and I fell asleep thinking of her. When I woke up, I buzzed for her to bring me my blood results. Trish handed me the paper printout. I glanced at the small page. White blood cells…300. Jen was right. "Trish, my white cells are 300. That's normal!"

"I know, I saw earlier. That's good news!"

A normal blood count meant I was slowly recovering from a bone marrow transplant, something that many people aren't fortunate enough to do. But I couldn't be happy about it because it was also a sign that my physical super powers, at least, were gone. I wasn't extraordinary any more. The awesome recovery that I was able to stage while I was battling Ewing's was not happening this time. As far as I could tell, I wasn't recovering, avoiding problems or surviving any more easily or faster than other patients. I was just an ordinary bone marrow transplant patient. But I was surviving and surviving was all I cared about. I was okay with being normal. Maybe it was time to pass the Super-Jew tee shirt on to someone who needed it.

My dad has a more predictable life than anyone I know. He walks at least four miles every day and has eaten the same lunch at work for the past fifteen years. Every Sunday during football season, he drinks a cream soda sometime between 2:00 and 3:00, no sooner, no later. After my transplant, every day was exactly like the previous day.

Even though to most people my life was a loll in a big bed in a sterile room with nothing much going on, I e-mailed Nick and Terry daily with details of my progress. I felt like they had gone through the transplant with me. I sent Nick the NC-17 version of my transplant stories, and Terry the watered-down, PG-13 versions. For instance, I told Nick a problem was "horrible" whereas I cleaned the description up to "pretty bad" when I wrote to Terry. I wouldn't allow myself to ever complain to Terry, even in e-mails, but sometimes I went off-course with Nick.

He was so great as a listener that I could exempt myself from the No Complaining Rule occasionally when I wrote to him.

Generally speaking, I was in a constant feverish state, which was fairly normal but still taken seriously. My new marrow repopulated very slowly, leaving my immune system open to virtually every disease in the world. Fevers could be caused by GVHD, infection, or the body's response to the growth of new bone marrow. The brightest transplant doctors in the world with access to the best technology sometimes can't determine the cause.

When the skin is inflamed, it can't function properly. One thing the skin does is regulate the body's temperature. Skin can become less able to retain water, thus becoming dry. My malfunctioning skin and constant fevers made me cold all the time, even when I wore heavy warm-up pants, thick socks, and a hooded sweatshirt. I bundled under five blankets. I had to psych myself up before getting out of bed. It felt like switching between a cool tropical night and the liquid nitrogen tank where my sperm is stored. Once I crawled back under the blankets, it took six minutes to stop shivering.

My calves were covered with white flakes. The GVHD specialist had me get a skin biopsy, but the results were inconclusive. Discovering the cause of a rash is not a scientific process. "Skin appears to be consistent with graft vs. host disease, but no evidence of GVHD could be found." When skin docs don't know what to call an ailment, they identify it as "nonspecific dermatitis." That means anything and everything and nothing.

Shortly after graduating from Virginia Tech, Jonathan flew to Minneapolis to stay with us. My mom had wanted to fly back East to watch him walk, but Jonathan had told her that he was going to skip the ceremony and play golf instead. Once he arrived, he bought a membership to the University of Minnesota gym and found a job delivering bag lunches to offices downtown. I loved having him around, and I think my

parents did too. They would never admit it, but staying with me was a chore. Having Jonathan gave them as much of a break as it did me.

Jonathan brought the remainder of his DVDs, leaving us with close to 200. My nurses gasped at the sight of our movie collection. We had one tower of thirty-five DVDs, as well as two rows spanning the length of the long windowsill. "You guys have got your own Blockbuster," Jen said with appreciation. At least half of them were comedies, because I always benefitted from a laugh. I loved the action adventures of Jerry Bruckheimer who has said, "We are in the transportation business. We transport audiences from one place to another." His movies certainly took me out of my sterile room. One of my favorite DVDs, *Speed,* took me on a roaring bus down LA freeways and up Sandra Bullock's skirt. There are few actors more talented than Keanu Reeves.

But even with all those movies to watch, I dreaded the hundred days ahead. I finally was allowed to leave my room because my white blood cells had been steadily climbing for a week. When they reached 1,200, I tightened the particulate mask around my nose and stepped outside my door to roam the halls.

My destination was the back corner seating area where I could flip through the magazines, hoping to get aroused. I felt free, even though I was confined to the fourth floor and chained to my IV pole. My parents always wanted to join me on my walks, but I wouldn't let them.

I paused in front of patient rooms to look at the photographs of the young children and their families. I read the material posted on the bulletin boards. I peered into the nurse's lounge hoping to glimpse what kind of takeout Jen was eating that day. I greeted the nurses. Once I got to the back corner, I settled in with the fashion magazines, hoping that one of the cute girls in the ads would be enough to get wood. This was the only time in the hospital that my mind was clear enough to get an actual erection.

I normally preferred the company of others, but there's something

to be said about solitude. I didn't have to think about how my parents might scrutinize my facial expressions. No one was monitoring my behavior: "Benjamin isn't sighing today, there must be something wrong. We have to tell the doctor," they might whisper.

As it turned out, my white blood cells did recover quickly. The white cells were resilient, too. Once they reached a mark, they rarely dipped back down, as was the case for most other patients. Maybe my super powers just needed a break, like my parents did.

For breakfast I ate a small bowl of Froot Loops. For lunch I ate my mom's tuna salad—tuna, celery, mayonnaise, egg white and sweet pickle. For dinner I ate grapes and strawberries. It was a step up from the ice chips and crackers I had been consuming for the past month.

The only true way to appreciate food is when it's taken away from you for a fucking month. What I went through was no Yom Kippur fast, which by the way, before cancer, I could only do once. Even then, I cheated by eating spearmint Tic Tacs throughout the day. This was a daily bombardment of incurable famishment. I got used to the pain, but the desire to taste was overwhelming.

When I told Jonathan to pick up a plain cheese pizza from Domino's and put it in the refrigerator, he said, "If you're going to eat pizza for the first time, don't you want it to be special, as in, not from Domino's? Also, why would you want it cold?"

"I want to start with what I know, and I know Domino's. And I'm afraid that hot food will make me throw up."

Jonathan delivered pizza for Domino's for six years of winter and summer breaks. This was before the time of GPS navigation systems, but he didn't need one. Jonathan has always been good with directions that his nickname could be Garmin. He'd always bring home free pizzas, which I loved. Ultimately, he consumed so many that he became averse to Domino's the way I was to salmon.

So I ate one slice of cold pizza, one more the next day and one-

and-a-half pieces warmed up two days later as we watched Final Destination. Jonathan and I both agreed that I could temporarily live on a diet of pizza.

The downside of being able to retain food was that I now had to take my medication orally. I was horrible at taking pills, so I had my nurse cut acyclovir, an antiviral medication, into fours. I crushed my Bactrim, an antibiotic used to prevent a dangerous form of pneumonia called PCP, into applesauce. I took twenty-two small pills of cyclosporine, my immunosuppressant. Counting all the increments, my nine medications approached a daily pill count of sixty.

My first solid shit was a mishmash of brown and orange. Alarmed, I asked my nurse Melissa Graver why. She explained. "For a while your poop may resemble the color of the food you ate." Melissa had actually requested the job of being one of my primary nurses because I reminded her of her teenage son. Although being older and a mom and all, she wasn't as hot as Jen and Trish, she gave me more affectionate care than they did. She always answered questions honestly, so my parents cherished her too. I could almost forgive her for being a huge NASCAR fan.

Melissa loved to gossip. Another one of her patients was an eight-year-old boy. She let him know all about me, and taught him to look up to me as a role model. She told me that for his Transplant Day gift, the hospital had given him a remote-controlled Hummer. As soon as he was allowed to leave his room, this boy revved up his Humvee and drove it down the hallway in the hopes of catching a glimpse of me through my window. As he passed, I tried to radiate some of my super powers. I wanted him to sense the strength emanating from my soul. As I went into my second month, I could feel that strength returning.

Most cancer patients have a secretary in the family who keeps others apprised of their progress. My mom kept fifty friends and relatives abreast of my health through weekly e-mails. I told her I thought reporting on me as though I were a war was a revolting act, but, according

to her, it was one that had to be done. "If I don't write bulletins, then people ask how you are. This way, I don't have to respond to fifty different e-mails."

She had to write them, but I didn't have to read them. Jonathan would check with me after he got her bulletins to make sure Mom's exaggerations were unfounded. He read one aloud to me. It was over 700 words long and used the phrase, "not out of the woods" twice. The person she referred to as Benjamin wasn't really me, but rather some other teenager about to die. The reality she described was far-off from the one I believed I was in. With her dramatic mother love, she entertained a worst-case scenario, whereas I felt my life depended on an unswerving belief that I would survive, no matter what came my way.

I was finally starting to feel better just when farm-fresh fruits were hitting the markets. Of all the foods I could have eaten, it was fruit that I wanted most. I couldn't stop thinking about how amazing it would taste: how the juice would burst out of the skin on my first bite, and how I would let it run down my chin. I would sink my teeth into the flesh, slowly, and allow it to melt on my tongue. When there was nothing left, I would suck on the pit until I was ready for the next piece.

A nice man who volunteered to assist patients' families brought me a basket of plums, nectarines and peaches. I didn't sleep at all the night he delivered them because I was so excited about eating these luscious fruits. But when I woke up in the morning, my tongue had deep ridges and was covered in thick yellow yeast as fuzzy as those ripe, round peaches. A CT scan revealed that I had sinusitis.

I tried hard just to sniff the nectarine, but I couldn't. I was crushed. I felt like all the progress I had made in getting back to a normal diet had been wiped out. Even though I couldn't taste or smell anything, the basket kept me dreaming; it gave me hope for the future, for a time when I would taste the wonderful fruit. The experience was not fruitless, after all.

A few days later, I noticed tiny red pieces floating in my urinal after peeing. I called a nurse.

"Oh, these are just specks of blood, "she said.

"Blood?" I was terrified.

"We see it all the time," she said.

What wasn't normal around here? I wondered. Later, when they got bigger, I called her back again. "Look, the pieces are bigger. They're not specks any more."

"They can get pretty big," she said. "I've seen some that are the size of half-dollars."

My dried blood progressed to a more unnerving form, hemorrhagic cystitis. My urine turned red. The first time it came spurting out of my penis, I stared fascinated at the urinal, unable to look away. Dr. Fry, who was big on explaining things, told me that I had an inflammatory bladder condition stemming from the BK virus. Eighty percent of the population carries a latent form of this virus but mine had settled in my kidneys after the transplant. . Each bloody piss contained at least one clot. Some were small and passed without me noticing. The painful ones were large and briefly stalled the urine flow.

Later that week, I woke up in the middle of the night needing to urinate. As I stood next to my bed, pulling my boxers down with my right hand and holding the urinal with my left, I contracted my detrusor muscle to squeeze out urine. After half-a-second of consistent stream, the urine flow ceased. I tried to pee again, but only a few drops fell.

I rushed into the bathroom. In the bright light, I looked through the clear plastic and saw that the liquid inside resembled not bloody urine, but thick red blood. A clot had broken away from my bladder and blocked the urethral orifice.

I tried peeing from different locations and positions. If you didn't know better, you'd think I was practicing for another visit to the sperm

bank. I gave up after an hour and summoned Melissa.

"I can't pee. I think there's a huge clot," I said.

"How bad do you need to go?"

"It's bad. I've been trying to pee for an hour. I think I need to be catheterized."

"Okay. I'll get someone to help you."

I felt intense pressure in my bladder, much like the time when I couldn't pee after surgery. I wondered if my bladder would explode. Melissa came in with a male nurse, a supposed expert at catheterization. He inserted the straight catheter and drained me. When he removed it, he said that my clots could have been jolted enough for me to pee them out. "What if they don't come out?" I asked.

"Then we do this again."

"They better fucking come out," I thought to myself. My next pee was going fine for a few seconds, and then the urine flow was once again stalled. Then wham! A half-dollar size clot pushed through my penis and into the container. I do believe it read: In Ben's penis we trust.

As soon as that problem cleared up, there was a new one. Results from CT scans of my head and lungs were terrible: I had infections in both mastoid bones, as well as in one of my lungs. Dr. Fry said he had to assume it was the highly dangerous Aspergillus fungus which, when it infects the lungs, has a mortality rate of at least fifty percent. He wanted to start me on Abelcet, which can cause kidney damage.

Melissa started my Abelcet around 4:30 p.m., and my dad and brother left shortly after to eat dinner and then go to the Metrodome to see the Twins play the Rockies. Even though my mom would get mad at them for leaving, they would attend a game every week sitting in the seven-dollar section. I didn't mind at all. I would be sitting right next to them if I could have. I think the part of those evenings my dad enjoyed most was eating food that wasn't from the hospital. Since I despised hospital food, he ate my lunch and dinner—the same five or six dishes over and

over again—every day. After he had downed over 150 hospital meals, he remarked, "I'd have no problem eating prison food after this."

After they left, I started one of my favorite movies, *Dumb & Dumber,* and that's when things went haywire. At first I was chilled and asked for a warm blanket. Then I began to shiver. Minutes later I was shaking. "Benjamin, what's the matter?" my mom asked.

"I don't know. I'm really cold."

Mom called in Melissa. "It's a reaction to Abelcet," Melissa said. "We can only stop it by giving Benjamin medication. I'm sure he will be okay. Let me check on that med." Her voice was calm but she darted out of the room faster than an okapi in the path of a leopard.

As the minutes ticked by, my shaking grew worse. Every muscle in my body wanted to convulse. I was freezing, but no amount of blankets, hides or blubber could warm me. When my teeth started to chatter, Mom said, "I'll be right back." This time I didn't mind her tendency to exaggerate my problems: I could hear her telling Melissa that I was on the verge of a grand mal seizure.

The two of them were at my side in seconds. Melissa kneeled next to my bed. "Ben, listen to me carefully. You're not going to have a seizure, I promise. Abelcet sometimes causes severe reactions, and I have already informed the attending. We've ordered Decadron. Have you had that before?"

"No."

"It's a steroid that will stop the reaction. I should have told you this could happen earlier, but I didn't want to scare you. The second I get the Decadron, I'll be right back here. I know you're scared, but you will not have a seizure. Do you understand?"

"Yes."

Melissa rushed out to secure Decadron. My shaking had become violent, causing my mattress to bounce up and down. "What can I do? Tell me what to do!" my mom shouted at me. My teeth were chattering

and the bed was squeaking, so I could hardly hear her.

"I can't stop shaking, "I shouted back. "I just wish I could stop shaking."

After forty minutes of this madness, Melissa burst in with a large syringe full of Decadron. "This may make you nauseous, so be prepared."

"I don't care. Please make it stop."

Melissa pushed the steroid into my Hickman and the shaking subsided. Nausea took its place. I puked once, and minutes later I puked again. I finished watching *Dumb & Dumber* as my body reacted to the shaking, causing my temperature to rise to 102.1 degrees. I stayed in bed motionless for the rest of the evening, drifting in and out of consciousness.

My dad and brother stopped by my room after the game. "Who won?" I asked.

"The Twins lost five to nothing," my dad replied. "But Torii Hunter made an amazing catch. You should have seen it! He leaped over the wall to rob this guy of a homerun. He must've jumped five feet in the air."

"Yeah, well, you missed the nightmare Benjamin just went through," my mom said. She was making my dad feel guilty for being absent.

"Too bad I won't be able to see it on *SportsCenter,*" I said, interrupting my mom. "Tell Dad what happened to me later if you want, I don't care. All of you get out, I'm going to bed."

In my hospital room, if I lowered my hand in the air, or simply said, "Stress level," then my family quieted down. I would have liked to have had that rule implemented throughout my childhood. I hated it when my parents used my situation to snipe at each other. I wondered how cancer had changed their relationship. I knew they had stopped watching TV together in the evenings sometime after I started going to NIH. I worried that once I got healthy, they would have less to talk about.

I received Abelcet for nearly a month, after I had been pre-medicated with the steroid hydrocortisone to prevent reactions like the one I had

with the first dose. With that experience behind me, I concentrated on my survival. When my next-door neighbor got a nasty lung infection, I asked Melissa: "Can I contract his infection?"

"No," she said curtly, appalled by my insensitivity.

"But his space is a cesspool," I pointed out to her. "Not only does he vomit thirty times a day, he has an infection!"

"You have nothing to worry about."

I let it go but I couldn't help noticing that his nurses were covered head to toe before entering, and stripped their outer layers after exiting. He was like their transmissible pet monkey. Since Melissa would not gossip with me about this guy, I tried to pump my dad for information. "What exactly is wrong with him?" I asked.

"How should I know? I don't ask too many questions."

Melissa didn't stay mad at me for long which was a good thing because my other nurse Jen was leaving for an assignment in England. She was going to care for a baby who would soon receive a transplant. Jen was only three years older than me. If we had met in different circumstances, I would have been too timid to talk to her—she was much too pretty. When I heard she was leaving, my fantasies began. If I ask you to marry me will you stay? We can produce as many babies as my frozen sperm allows…and then we can continue trying long after that. Without Jen, the hospital would be a lot less fun.

For a month, my doctors had been saying I would be released soon. But every time my departure seemed possible, a new health problem would arise. It began to feel like a higher power was forcing me to stay. One time I spiked a fever the very morning I was supposed to leave. I was permitted to go outside and take a walk, or sit on one of the hospital benches, but I wouldn't do it. My mom couldn't understand why. Perhaps cancer's greatest gift is the apperception that when human desire is left unfulfilled for long stretches of time and then is finally realized, the joy proves to be worth the wait. I wanted the day I was released to

be the sweetest redemption of all, and I didn't want to diminish it with pointless breaths of fresh air.

Thursday, June 19 was the day the docs said I could leave. My punishment had been sixty-five consecutive days in the hospital, so my reward would be great. I had forgotten what the world looked like without peering through glass. There was nothing that would stop me from leaving.

My dad and brother had already packed my things, including my Rocky poster, and taken them to the apartment. I peed one last time before leaving. After a long absence, my hemorrhagic cystitis had returned.

Trish was the first to console me. "I'm so sorry, Ben. You deserve to go home."

"Is there any way I can leave?"

"Only if your urine clears up."

I drank water and waited. One hour later it was time to pee again. I said a short prayer. God must have heard me because my urine was crystal clear.

Dr. Fry had made sure that I knew to stay cautious. I read over the transplant unit's discharge material, which was a less intense version of NIH's "Benjamin can die this many ways." Report all symptoms ranging from uncontrolled bleeding to fatigue. Stay away from people, plants and construction sites. Wear a particulate mask at all times when away from the apartment. My release from Room 210 was not a license to rebel. The attending signed the discharge form, and I put on my shoes and particulate mask. I walked out the door and down the corridor. "Don't forget to come back and visit us!" Trish yelled from the nurse's desk. I was going to miss her.

My mom and I rode the elevator down, walked past the hospital lobby and through the automatic doors. A revolving door and five feet stood between me and the world. I paused to think about what I had just accomplished.

TWICE

Last time I had survived exposure to K-Metal in the form of chemo. This time the kryptonite that threatened my powers had come like a meteor from an exploded planet in outer space. I had no impenetrable skin or super bone marrow to protect me. There was only modern medicine and highly skilled doctors and nurses to sustain me. Now I understood what other Sick Kids like Alexis had gone through, how making it to the other side can be a struggle, a tug-of-war with not only cancer, but also with hope.

I entered the revolving door, pushed it all the way around and stepped onto the concrete outside. It was four in the afternoon on a warm afternoon with gray, low-hanging clouds smothering the sun. A calm breeze touched my face. I lifted my particulate mask off and pulled in a slow, deep breath. The leaves had never looked greener, and the world had never looked clearer. This was the single happiest moment in my life. Certainly there will be other happy times—perhaps my wedding, the birth of my child, my book being published—and all of them will be compared to this Thursday afternoon and will ultimately come up short because my mind has elevated it to an unreachable height.

At the apartment, I listened to a song I couldn't get out of my head: Travis Tritt's "It's a Great Day to be Alive." I wasn't angry that I had gotten a second cancer when I was nineteen, or that I had been poked and prodded every which way, or that I had lived in a single hospital room without ESPN for more than two months. I felt like the most fortunate person in the world. I would give my big left nut now just to experience the exhilaration of that afternoon again. The next day, I confided to Terry in an e-mail that I was getting ready for the ultimate digestion test:

> I realize I'm going to sound like a chick, but I'll say it anyway. I have a new respect for life. Small things, too, like the color of the trees outside my window. Or the smell and taste of food. My mom bought me Cinnabon today. Or the taste of air. Yeah, you can taste it if you try hard enough.

These cinnamon rolls are so unhealthy you might as well inject fat straight into your vein. It's also one of the best-tasting foods on the planet, and I wanted one.

I began to nibble on the huge pastry, and thirty minutes later I had eaten three-quarters of it. I went back to my La-Z-Boy, happy with my digestive accomplishment. But I started to feel sick. I couldn't eat anything for the rest of the day.

I hoped to sleep off the nausea, but I woke-up with an acute pain in my lower back and took two Tylenol. Had my liver exploded from the Cinnabon? Before I could crawl back into bed, I felt that familiar urge, grabbed my bucket and barfed.

But Ben, you haven't eaten anything for hours. What could you have vomited? The wretched smell told the whole story. I had thrown up the Cinnabon that I had attempted to digest eight hours earlier. My stomach had been unable to push the Cinnabon into my intestine. I told Jonathan that I didn't want any more Cinnabons and that he could eat the rest of the box. "If I ate all those it would kill me," he said.

The chemo hadn't killed me. The radiation hadn't killed me. The lung fungus hadn't killed me, but I had almost gotten done in by a cinnamon roll.

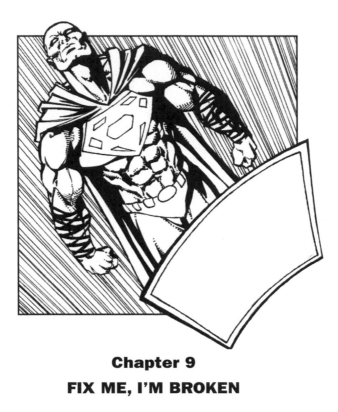

Chapter 9
FIX ME, I'M BROKEN

Caution: This section may make you queasy. Proceed at your own risk.

3:30 a.m.: I stagger into the bathroom and pull my penis out through the slit in my boxers. The hydration pump attached to my Hickman like a Siamese twin is set at 200 milliliters per hour to prevent blood clots. It also wakes me up every two hours to pee. I begin urinating and three bloody drips later, I freak. Oh, no. Don't do this to me again.

3:31 a.m.: I move around hoping to dismember the blood clots. I try peeing again. Not a single drip. I know right away there's a big mother-fucker in there.

3:32 a.m.: I tiptoe into my parents' bedroom and wake my dad. "What is it, Benjy?" he asks.

"You need to call the hospital, I need to be admitted. I can't pee."

"Are you sure? Why don't you try again?"

"No, I tried twice. I need to go immediately."

4:20 a.m.: Forty-five minutes after my dad called, an escort van picks us up and drops us at the hospital.

4:25 a.m.: On arriving at the transplant unit, my nurse takes me to my new room adjacent to my old one, Room 211. "Who's is in my old room?" I ask.

"Oh, that's your old neighbor. He got discharged just like you, but returned yesterday."

My new room is much smaller. My white board reads "Welcome Back Ben!"

5:00 a.m.: I really have to urinate. At least my nurse has paused my hydration pump.

5:25 a.m.: I originally ask for morphine, but when my nurse tells me it'll take an hour for the order to arrive, instead ask for a 25-milligram dose of Benadryl. Damn, that drug has a million uses.

5:30 a.m.: Two nurses enter my room to give me a straight catheter. My penis is like Kobe Bryant—always needing a double-team. My bladder is bursting and I'm wondering where else the fluid can go. Is it possible to backtrack into my kidneys?

5:32 a.m.: One of the nurses slowly pushes the white plastic tube into my penis and through my urethral sphincter. Dark red liquid streams out the tube and into the pink spit bucket.

6:30 a.m.: Time to pee again. I assume half-dollar size clots will push through, however only drips of blood find their way out. Nurse, could you please shove that tube up my dick again?

7:00 a.m.: My nurse inserts the second straight catheter.

8:00 a.m.: I try to urinate, and again I'm unsuccessful. It's obvious that something is really wrong.

8:30 a.m.: Melissa wants to insert a larger, more permanent catheter

which has two ends. The longer end feeds into a collection bag. "We're going to try to break up the clot through this shorter end," Melissa says.

"What do you mean, 'break up?'"

"I'm going to fill a large syringe with sterile water and slowly push it into your bladder. Then I'm going gently pull on the syringe. Hopefully, the clot will break up and be sucked into the syringe."

8:40 a.m.: I can feel the water filling my bladder accompanied by a strong urge to pee, and then a slow emptying as Melissa draws it back. She pulls out some clots. Afterward, my urine flows nicely through the catheter.

10:00 a.m.: The collection bag is filling slowly, and my bladder is accumulating urine. "What's happening?" I ask Melissa.

"I don't know. The attending just ordered an ultrasound to see what's going on."

10:30 a.m.: The ultrasound technician wheels a large, portable ultrasound machine into my room. She places the transducer probe on my bladder and we look at the screen. "What exactly are we looking at?" I ask.

"That's your bladder. And that small circle is the balloon from the end of the catheter."

"What's all that stuff on the bottom of my bladder?"

"That...is...your...blood clot."

"That's impossible. That thing is one-third the size of my bladder."

11:00 a.m.: "We're going to try something different," the attending doctor says to me.

"What is it? I have already had three catheters and would appreciate if I only get one more."

"The head urologist will try to remove the clot through a special catheter. We think that'll work."

"What if it doesn't?"

"Then you may need surgery on your bladder."

12:00 p.m.: A scowling, big-headed woman enters my room with a

goody bag. "This is the catheter I'm going to use," she says, pointing to a tube wide enough to wrap around my dick.

"You're kidding, right? You're going to stick that in my penis?"

"Yes. I have to warn you—this is not going to be fun." I try to mentally induce a speedy release of endorphins. Zillions and zillions of endorphins.

12:01 p.m.: "Ben, I've already ordered you morphine," Melissa says. "It should be here very shortly."

12:02 p.m.: The urologist explains the procedure. The catheter has six small holes at the penis-end. She is going to vigorously push sterile water into my bladder, and then suck it out. The clot will exit through the six holes. "Hopefully the holes don't clog," she says.

12:15 p.m.: After a morphine dose unworthy of a penis problem as minimal as chafing, the insanity begins. I squeeze Melissa's hand and smother my face with my pillow. The manic urologist shoots a large syringe of water into my bladder, and yanks it back. Tons of stringy blood clots fill the syringe. "It's working," she says, emptying the clots out of the syringe, ready to go again. The urologist is punishing my bladder and it feels like aqua blue fire repeatedly exploding through my genitalia.

12:20 p.m.: "Ben, are you breathing?" Melissa asks.

"Yeah, I'm breathing."

"Just keep breathing, I'm right here."

12:30 p.m.: I break out in hysterics. "Is something wrong?" Melissa asks. "And why are you laughing?"

"I don't know what else to do." I have only two options, to laugh or cry. What is happening to my penis? Old Benito gets too little notice as it is.

12:45 p.m.: The urologist is finally done taking her anger out on my poor bladder and most of my clot is gone. She removes the monster penile catheter and inserts the fifth and final tube, a three-way Foley

catheter. This one is permanent.

12:50 p.m.: Melissa brings in a tall pole with six three-liter bags of water hanging from the top. The bags all drain into my bladder through one of my catheter's three compartments, and the residual fluid exits through another. This tube is long, traveling across my floor and ending at the shower drain. This is known as continuous bladder irrigation, and its purpose is to prevent blood clots.

With my family, I watch the color inside the tube change from red to light red. I have lost considerable blood through my bladder, which means I will have to receive more platelet and red blood cell transfusions. I don't eat, drink, flinch or peep. Never again will I have five penile catheters inserted in a seven-and-a-half hour stretch of time.

My bladder bled and bled and bled. The color flowing through the tube was dark pink, but became bright red if I wiggled, coughed or vomited. Over a hundred liters of sterile water flowed in and out of me. Ironically, the patient next to me also developed hemorrhagic cystitis and was on continuous bladder irrigation. Why did we keep getting the same ailments? Since our rooms were next to each other, dozens of water bags were piled between our doors. In a fucked up way, I found that funny. I wasn't absolutely sure that Melissa wasn't shitting me when she told me I would not contract any of his infections.

I stopped eating because vomiting caused bladder irritation and painful spasms. I left the bed only once each day. My mom arranged a chair, bucket of hot water and a washcloth one foot from my bed. After I cleaned myself, I slithered around the halls as my dad pushed my IV and irrigation poles. My stride was short because big steps tugged at my catheter. What once had been my joyous hour of freedom had now become the worst part of my day. Shuffling around in my hospital gown, with a tube leading from my penis to a bag full of blood while my dad pushed my poles, was the most degrading experience of my life. My

parents, doctors, and nurses ordered me to move about. "You can get pneumonia or a blood clot in your leg," they had said.

One night, I developed another clot that blocked the catheter. For the next four hours, Trish manually irrigated my bladder through the third compartment of the Foley catheter. "In order to remove the clot, we may need to replace the catheter," the attending said.

"Do whatever is necessary to dislodge the clot, but this catheter isn't coming out."

Finally, two six-inch long clots traveled across the floor and into the shower drain. This same incident occurred continuously over the coming days. My ability to retain food vanished, and I restarted TPN. Most of my meds were switched back to IV form. I atrophied from lying motionless for twenty-three hours each day. I was so miserable that I wouldn't check my e-mails until my mom forced me. I watched TV or slept constantly. The catheter would be removed when the fluid flushed out of my bladder was consistently light pink. Too bad it was as crimson as a rose.

My single joy that week was watching Arnold Schwarzenegger movies with my dad in honor of the release of *Terminator 3: Rise of the Machines*. We were angry when Arnold became governor and stopped making movies. Like Rocky and Superman, he could take my mind off my misery, including my inability to digest anything, even a small bowl of cereal.

I didn't want anyone to see me in this condition but this was the moment when Aunt Elsa decided to visit with my adorable cousins. I knew Elsa's visit would cheer up my mom so I agreed to let them come to my room even though I felt sick. "I don't feel so good," I announced to them after twenty minutes. "I think I'm gonna throw up."

Aunt Elsa didn't get the message to leave. I leaned forward, opened my mouth wide and spewed into my bucket. Aunt Elsa and her girls

held their ground, pretending not to be bothered. My eleven-year-old cousin Emma, sitting inches away from me, wiped her face to make sure none of the crispy rice flakes sprayed her, and smiled. I'm sure I must have scarred her for life.

A few days later, the urologist came into my room. "It's time to remove the catheter," he said.

"Are you sure? What if I develop another big clot?"

"You have to give it a shot. We can't leave it in any longer."

I went eighteen consecutive days with a tube in my penis, which was eighteen more days of attention than it normally received. Although I was afraid that I would be re-catheterized immediately, I couldn't take it anymore. This "nuisance," as some of my doctors labeled my condition, was crippling my body and spirits. It tested my No Complaining rule, my superiority to sadness and everything else my Super Man complex induced.

Trish deflated the catheter balloon and gently pulled out the tube. I looked down, but quickly looked back up. "What the fuck is that?"

Trish looked at it and said, "I don't know." Then she asked another nurse if it was normal for the tip to look like it was growing a Bubblicious bubble. "That's common. It'll go back to normal," Trish said.

I dressed in my favorite yellow Adidas pants as I planned my next pee. I would wait exactly one hour to ensure that I had collect enough urine to create pressure, but not long enough for huge clots to develop.

Precisely one hour later, I walked into the bathroom and closed the door behind me. I even prayed: "Dear God: Please help me pee right now. I'll do anything for You. Anything You ever ask me to do, I'll do it, I promise. If You want me to stop drinking alcohol for the rest of my life, I'll do it. Just please, please grant me this one wish that I wish right now. Dear God: please help me pee. Amen."

I grabbed the plastic urinal and dropped my pants. I pulled in a deep

breath as I slowly felt some bladder pressure. I released and got two drip. "Oh, God help me." Half a second later, I saw three more drips…then boom! A cube-shaped clot burst through and nailed the bottom of the urinal with a thud. A tiny trickle of blood, and then a second cube hit the urinal like Dustin Diamond's career. Finally, I was free-flowing. "Thank you, God."

"I peed," I said, and my parents and brother congratulated me. For the rest of the day, I urinated every forty-five minutes on the dot. When I napped in the afternoon, I told Jonathan to wake me at exactly 3:30 so I could pee. My pee was bloody with some small clots. That night I told my nurse to wake me up every forty-five minutes. "I might roll back over and fall asleep, so hit me if you have to. Do not let me go back to sleep," I ordered her.

She neglected to wake me once. Fortunately, I stirred thirty minutes later and passed some large clots. I continued this forty-five minute sequence for over a week, even though my urine mostly cleared a few days later.

For the next two months, I pissed some blood each day. In mid-September, I went to the ER to be catheterized because of a blockage. Two days later, my urine completely cleared and I haven't seen a trace of blood since, even though Dr. Fry said that my hemorrhagic cystitis could return weeks, months, or even years later.

Dr. Fry stated that he had never seen such a quick recovery before. My parents attributed it to the prayers of my family and friends (my mom gave updates on my bleeding organ and asked people to pray for it.) I chalked it up to just another random event. While it was still bleeding, some urologists had mentioned using toxic chemicals to patch my bladder. "I think I'll wait and see what happens," I had told them.

I joked with Jonathan that I should have kept a Junk Count right alongside my Puke Count. Not even Wilt Chamberlain had as many

people see his package in such a short period of time.

It was much easier to enjoy beautiful Minneapolis away from the hospital. I walked instead of riding in the escort van for my clinic appointments. On many afternoons, Jonathan and I walked to Blockbuster down the street. I guess our 200 DVDs weren't enough. I was embarrassed wearing my particulate mask in public, but sometimes you just have to say "fuck it."

My mom became friends with a woman who worked for the Minnesota Twins. She set us up in a secluded press box for two games. In the sixth inning of the first game, the jumbo screen read, "Special welcome to Benjamin Rubenstein. You are awesome! Hang in there!"

We got the privilege to meet Harmon Killebrew, who spoke with us in the press box for twenty minutes. Harmon had been inducted into the National Baseball Hall of Fame in 1984 and at the time was sixth on the all-time homerun leaders list with 573 homers. At the age of sixty-seven, he still looked like he could knock a couple out of the park. He signed a ball for me, which still sits in a trophy case in my bedroom.

I also acquired a Vikings hat signed by the quarterback Daunte Culpepper, who in 2004, had the fourth highest passer rating of all time, and a paper autographed by the Vikings' Chris Hovan, Michael Bennett, Daunte Culpepper, and Randy Moss, one of the best wide receivers ever. The paper reads, "Ben—you've cheered for us, now we're cheering for you. Go Vikes!" I also corralled a bobblehead of Goldy Gopher, the delightful University of Minnesota mascot.

I would later get an autographed picture of Frank Howard, the two-time American League Home Run King, and a football signed by Marcus Allen, then the eighth leading rusher in NFL history. Finally, the baseball from Lou Brock's 3000th hit completed my Minnesota collection. He'd signed it, of course. All of these collectibles were added to my

Wall of Fame. If I could only have gotten The Bachelor's autograph, my life would have been complete.

Dr. Fry discontinued my TPN for the second time and I was expected to maintain my weight. I documented everything I consumed, which averaged 1,300 calories, which wasn't enough. Dr. Fry prescribed an appetite stimulant called Marinol, which is a synthetic version of THC, the psychoactive component of marijuana. "This might give you the munchies," he said.

Marinol was exciting because I was eating more and had a crucial buzz. One afternoon after swallowing the small circular pill, I saw a bulge in my lower gum in the mirror. A small bug had burrowed under the tissue and was wriggling. Blood was dripping down my chin. I asked Jonathan if he saw it, too. "What the hell are you talking about?" he said.

I was hallucinating. I watched TV, terrified to move, worrying about everything. I was nervous that if I stepped away for any reason, even to pee, something bad might happen. I started playing *Madden* until Joey Porter jumped through the TV to get me. I threw the remaining Marinol pills in the trash after that, even though some friends offered money for them.

Even though I could barely eat, Jonathan drove me wherever I wanted to get food. I had to taste it all, no matter how few bites I could finish: curly fries, soft tacos with a thin layer of mild sauce, square thin crust pizza, a bacon cheeseburger, buttery popcorn, an ice cream strawberry shortcake, a large pretzel coated in salt and dripping with butter.

GVHD was on everybody's mind. I exhibited signs of Stage Two GVHD, fortunately without the liver problems, but a skin biopsy on my chest showed no evidence. Dr. Fry was concerned, and he preferred that I stay in Minnesota, but I twisted his arm to let me go home. It didn't hurt that my hundred day bone marrow biopsy results were fantastic.

I was far from healthy. My parents have a photo of me and Killebrew

that's tough to look at. My skin is pale and dry. My lips are swollen and peeling. My eyes, normally big and alive, looked exhausted. I'm wearing a hooded sweatshirt, even though it was July. That's not how I saw myself at the time, however. My Super Man complex would not allow me to see the reality.

My health was worsening; there was just no smoking gun to prove it. Even if I was approaching death, I had to return to Virginia sometime around the hundred day mark. That was the minimum, and staying longer meant other transplant patients were better than me. I accepted that I was normal, but I couldn't admit that I was inferior. I had to maintain hope that I was still a Super Man. The blood test that showed I had only 200 white blood cells and the penile catheter incident both tested my faith, but I didn't break.

After 122 days in Minnesota, my mom and I flew home. My dad and brother also embarked on their two-day road trip after transferring our possessions into the Big Red Box, including my sports memorabilia. I was happy to be going home, but I was also scared to leave.

Riding in the car through my neighborhood—the same one I lived in my whole life—the trees looked larger than I had remembered them. Terry told me Virginia got drenched with rain, and I could see the effects. I suddenly became nostalgic for the old days pre-cancer. I remembered from middle school riding my bike with Birdsall to the general store to buy candy. I pocketed the box to make sure it would fit, and the crazy store owner thought I was stealing and had called the cops.

I thought about the time soccer practice had been canceled because of rain. The trees had looked so big then, much like they did now. I thought all the way back to elementary school, when my friend and I had picked honeysuckle in front of his house. An even earlier memory was from kindergarten, when one of my best friends had moved away. I wondered if that's how my friends had thought of me, a friend who had

moved away. Andy and Drew had worked summer jobs at Don Pablo's along with another friend of ours. Worm and those three hung out just about every night. The new guy had replaced me. I had gone away, but now I was back. I was back for good.

I wanted to see some of my friends, so I called Andy, "Hey, I just got back. Do you have any food in your house?"

"Yeah man."

"Cool. You want to pick me up?"

"Sure."

My friends dubbed the summer before I was diagnosed with cancer in 2000 as "The Summer of Benjy." It was then that we bet who could last the longest without getting a job. Technically, my "job" was seeing films. I saw ten movies, most of them with Andy or Drew. Regal should have paid me to watch the movies.

I hung on to my traditional summer the way a woman with cancer clings to her last wisps of hair before chemo takes them all. My days had been carefree in the summers of my youth. My biggest concern was which friend I would hang out with, or whether we'd play Monopoly or pool. One year, I broke a window playing baseball, and Drew's parents had caught us watching the stripper scene from *True Lies*. I didn't get in much trouble for either.

I had yearned for a summer of old because I was slow to mature. I preferred traditional activities over age-appropriate ones, like earning money or hitting on girls. Most of my friends moved on, acting their age. Drew and Bently were the first out of the bet when they became lifeguards. Worm was next with his construction administration job, and Drew followed with his short stints as a Toys "R" Us employee and as a janitor, until he got fired.

In the summer of 2004, I conceded the victory to Nick once I became a guest service representative at Hollywood Video. I was a stellar

Hollywood Video employee. Several times I played a non-cartoon movie on the TVs that was not only frowned upon, but was blatantly against the rules. "But *Top Gun* is rated PG," I said. "I even fast forwarded the sex scene." There were anonymous complaints. I didn't know what the big deal was. *Top Gun* only used "shit" twenty-one times.

I received several odd requests, one from a small, Indian man in his fifties who said he wanted to ask me something. He then walked around the counter to the employee side, unbuckled the red rope that was meant to prevent these very incidents, and got very close to me, so close that I could smell his breath. He whispered, "Where's your porn, I know you got porn."

"We don't carry that here, but you might want to try Manassas Video Club. I've seen commercials." He left the store, but not before buckling the red rope.

During The Summer of Benjy, I developed a strong friendship with Andy, who I had known since I was four. We spent many afternoons rummaging for food in our kitchens, or at a fast food joint. Twice we went to Worm's house hoping his mom would fix us lunch. One time it worked, and the other time Worm kicked us out.

"We want food. What's your problem?" Andy asked.

"You guys show up at my house just so my mom will make you lunch," Worm said. "Does my house look like a restaurant? Get your own damn food."

Toward the end of The Summer of Benjy, my friends and I decided to buy cigars. Because of my He-Bro, semi-noticeable sideburns and chin fuzz, I looked the oldest and was forced to make the purchase. I walked into the store with sweat accumulating on my brow. After pretending to look around for ten minutes, I approached the counter.

"What can I do for you?" the employee asked.

"Yeah, let me get a pack of Black & Milds," I said in my deepest voice.

"Please don't card me," I was thinking.

"Sure thing."

I rushed out of the store as proud as could be. We all enjoyed our cigars on Andy's porch.

When Andy looked at me on this afternoon, I could tell I wasn't what he was expecting. It had only been three years since The Summer of Benjy, yet so much had changed. Andy saw a pasty, weakened kid connected to an IV hydration backpack wearing a particulate respirator mask. It was the same Benjy, just a little different on the outside.

We watched TV at his house and ate a Tombstone pizza that he cooked. I had one slice. After two hours, I felt tired and asked him to drive me home. I actually felt like the Sick Kid, and there was nothing I could do about it.

A few hours after Andy dropped me off, I developed a fever and headed to NIH. I had been home for only nine hours before being reminded I shouldn't have left Minneapolis. NIH had agreed to continue my post-transplant care, which was already scheduled to begin the next day, so I would simply be a little early.

My first CT scan, during the Summer of Benjy, showed clear lungs, but the one I received now didn't. "There's a spot in your lower left lung, the same place as your first fungal infection," Dr. Bruce said.

"Is it the same fungus?" I said.

"We don't know, and that's the reason we want to biopsy it. We need to know exactly what it is so we can treat it correctly. Because of the location, we can't give you conscious sedation. You're going to be awake for it."

On my way down, I passed Chief Levy. "Do you think it's the same fungus as I had in Minneapolis?" I asked.

"We don't know. Let's just hope it's fungus and not something else."

"Wait...you mean Ewing's?"

"We don't know, Ben."

Cancer recurrences are often more destructive than the original. My skin tingled with horror. I removed my shirt, stretched out on the table, and turned my head to the right. If I watched the needle pushing through my left lung, I would probably puke on the doctor's face. "I want you to take a breath and then exhale completely…now slowly inhale…stop right there."

I held my breath as the doctor forced the needle through my skin, in between two ribs, and into my left lung. It took him several attempts before completing the biopsy. The needle digging around my lung felt like warm bubbles rising to the surface and popping.

It wasn't cancer. I had a rare fungal infection called Fusarium, and was put on a new antifungal medication called voriconazole, which is much less toxic than the Abelcet I got in Minnesota. If voriconazole hadn't worked, then the next step would be to cut off part of my lung.

Nobody wants to face the possibility that he has cancer. But when it turns out to be a false alarm, the relief is unimaginable. Everybody who hears that they don't have cancer after all gains a powerful appreciation for life. Though the gratitude can be as brief as several minutes, it reminds you that any day is a great day to be alive.

The five or six blankets, even straight out of the hospital's incubator, weren't warming me. I wished a giant hen would sit on me. Or I could set myself on fire. I felt chilled at a hundred, cold at 101, and freezing at 102. At 103, there was no adjective in Webster's Dictionary to describe it.

My skin was inflamed from head to toe. I was supposed to slather myself with triamcinolone ointment, a topical steroid which would trap my body heat and make me feel warmer. But in order to use it, I had to get out of bed and away from the minimal warmth I had already established. I was in the Arctic and could either dive into the frozen lake

to reach the bear hide, or stay by the fire and hope that would suffice. It was one of my most difficult short-term decisions.

A staph infection in my Hickman caused my temperature hike. At 103.3, my temperature began to decline. I used the triamcinolone. I thought my bones would shatter while I shivered my way to the bathroom. The infection went away with the help of vancomycin, a powerful, broad-spectrum, last-resort antibiotic that I have received countless times over the years.

Dr. Bruce couldn't resolve what was wrong with my skin, the largest and most underrated organ of the human body. I went to Dermatology and stripped naked so doctors, nurses and even medical students could examine me. That wasn't unusual. In Minnesota no fewer than fifteen individuals saw my junk. What was weird was facing the wall, spreading my legs and bending down. I was in a different kind of prison, but the body cavity search remained.

After my recent cancer scare I felt that every day was a great day to be alive, except for the following two weeks when I stayed at NIH. I dealt with a Hickman infection, shingles, ankle swelling, elevated bilirubin and a high fever. When I expected to leave, the attending physician didn't want to release me because of my low potassium.

Potassium is a mineral that regulates the heartbeat and the activity of muscle tissue, and helps the kidneys function. Potassium deficiency can be dangerous. Through daily blood tests, NIH closely watched my level, while adding potassium to my IV hydration bags.

My potassium was 3.0 mEq/L while the normal range is between 3.5 and 5.0 mEq/L. Since my level was slowly creeping up, I weaseled my way into a discharge on the condition that I would receive IV potassium at home. Our local home health agency was faxed a prescription to put extra potassium into my hydration bags. I was surprised the attending physician was so concerned since my level was rising and barely below normal.

An employee at the home health agency delivered the hydration bags to our house. The man told me that the doctor had ordered such a high dose of potassium that he refused to administer it. He infused my hydration bags with half of the prescribed potassium, which was still far more than normal. "When you return to NIH, make sure your doctor checks your level. You don't want it getting too high," he said.

After that, the plan was to get my blood counts and then go home, but nothing was that simple at NIH. Jonathan bought me a pulled chicken sandwich, coleslaw and potato salad from the basement cafeteria. I ate a few bites before feeling full. Since leaving Minneapolis, I had lost some weight. My health seemed to decline on a daily basis. I spent most of my time at NIH, and I never had an appetite there. I became fearful about my future. I looked nothing like the muscled athletes I admired or even the kickers. I was wasting away.

Jonathan drove me to many of my checkups. We listened to "So Far Away" by Staind. I'm not good at understanding the meaning behind song lyrics, but to me the title said it all. I couldn't have been further away from my goal, with the exception of being dead. According to my health trend, I was on my way to the grave.

I was so far away from my beautiful university that Thomas Jefferson founded, and from the college life I was supposed to be living. I was so far away from my friends, who were accelerating past me not just in credit hours, but also in social experiences, maturity, and new friends, those tangible college credits.

The blood results took longer than usual. Jonathan and I reached the middle of our second movie when Dr. Bruce arrived. "Your potassium level came back elevated. Are you still getting potassium in your hydration bag?"

"Yeah."

"Press stop on the IV pump. We're going to take your blood one

more time."

"What was the number?"

"Yours is over eight, but normal is between three point five and five."

An hour after my second blood draw, an unfamiliar doctor appeared in his blue scrubs. "You need to come with me to the ICU right now. I have to get your potassium down."

Neither Jonathan nor I knew what was going on.

"I don't feel funny. What's the big deal?" I said.

"High potassium can cause lethal arrhythmias."

"So that's why we were rushing to a room containing every lifesaving device imaginable. My heart might stop," I thought.

I wasn't given the time to consider what was happening. I received injections of calcium and insulin to briefly counteract the potassium. The doctor thrust the two enormous vials into my Hickman, which caused a sensation of extreme warmth, like I had been shoved into a piping hot oven. "I feel really hot. Is this normal?"

"It'll go away soon."

I got an electrocardiogram, a test that records the electrical activity of the heart. The potassium had affected me because my T waves were tall.

The ICU doctor gave me Lasix to help me pee out the excess potassium. Then, he handed me a laxative drink. "You have to drink this as soon as you can," he said.

"All of it? I'm going puke it up."

"You have to drink it. If you throw it up then you have to try again."

I finished the putrid laxative, somehow without vomiting. What occurred over the next eight-and-a-half hours is something I would rather not remember. Let's just say that if I had kept a Shit Count, I would have blown away any and all competition.

My room's front wall was mostly glass and there were no curtains or blinds. The toilet was in a cubbyhole and barely out of view. Nurses

entered as they pleased. Before pooping, I told Jonathan to sit outside the door, face the opposite direction, and prevent anybody from entering. When I finished, I would yell at him to come back in.

At first the urge came every half hour, but by 9:00 p.m., I was shitting every ten minutes. I sometimes remained on the toilet, because I knew I would be back once I got to the bed. Meanwhile my fever was rising, because of my multiple infections, and I was freezing, dehydrated, exhausted and dizzy.

Jonathan stuck around until midnight, even though I kept saying he could leave. He would have stayed longer, but he had to open for Domino's in the morning. "Are you sure you'll be okay?" he asked.

"I'll be fine. I think the shitting is calming down."

At 3:00 a.m. a second electrocardiogram showed almost normal T waves. I resolved to never shit again. Just before I was transferred from the ICU to Floor 13, I saw my mom rush through the elevator and stop at the nurse's desk. "I want to speak with Dr. Trout right now!" She was trying to get the attending physician on the phone. "God help Dr. Trout," I thought. Nobody messes with my mom's two kids.

"Damn right you're sorry," my mom's voice echoed down the hall. "Ben went through hell last night. He could have died if the home health aide hadn't refused to give him the dose you prescribed."

There was a long silence when I imagined Dr. Trout who had always been pleasant and competent was defending herself.

"I'll be looking over your shoulder at everything you do," Mom told Dr. Trout. "You should be fired for what you did." Mom had the final word.

I felt like I was falling apart, so I requested Dr. Bruce to put me back on TPN. "I can't eat enough to maintain my weight."

"Ben, we wouldn't let that happen to you. TPN is hard on your organs. We want to keep you off it until it's absolutely necessary."

It was tough for me to look in the mirror, just as it was after my

haircut three years earlier when my curly locks had fallen to the barber shop floor. My muscles were tiny and soft, nothing like the firm fibers I had developed weightlifting at college. My shoulders slouched with the weight of my head. A meteor storm of kryptonite had assaulted me. I was fading into oblivion, and my super powers could not stop it.

My resolution never to shit again following the potassium incident in August lasted two weeks. The next week I felt mild, constant abdominal pain on my left side, which I thought was a strained muscle. Christine sent me for an X-ray, which showed a massive collection of excrement. "I have a quarter-mile back-up of shit," I told friends.

I ingested laxatives and stool softeners, and even took two suppositories. When I shoved the capsules up my ass, I closed my eyes, as if that would make any difference. Finally, small eruptions in my upper bowels pushed the shit through the winding corridors of my intestines—slowly, painfully and grotesquely. Through three days of frequent and long Shit-Capades, I cleaned house.

But I overdosed on laxatives, and on September 18, my relentless diarrhea arrived, along with Hurricane Isabel. News stations predicted many areas would lose power for days. No TV, PS2 or movies. What was I going to do—read? I wasn't sure I even remembered how.

Because our house was on a well and we were without electricity, each toilet could only be flushed once. But I was shitting several times each day, not to mention all those courtesy flushes. I refused to shit in a toilet that already has some shit in it.

My mom thought of one solution. She called around the neighborhood to see if anyone had water. "We need to transport buckets of water for Benjamin," she said.

"What does he need water for?" my neighbors asked.

"Well…he poops a lot and needs water to flush."

Our power returned, and no buckets were needed.

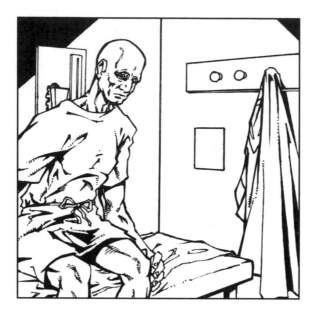

Chapter 10
MIRACLE JUICE

After the fiasco with Dr. Trout, I switched my care from NIH over to Dr. Jennsen at the Pediatric Hematology & Oncology Group of Northern Virginia. When I told Christine that I would transfer my transplant follow-up care to Dr. Jennsen, she understood. "I want you to do whatever makes you comfortable," she said.

NIH was directly associated with my cancer, one of the most significant events of my life, making it an equally important location to me. NIH consumed my time, and not just hours or days, but months. And not just a dot on the life span of the universe, or on one of the life spans of one of the universes, but the aging of my self. NIH brought me closer to life in the form of cancer freedom and closer to death by taking a portion of my aggregate heartbeats. NIH was like a living organism, not

a friend or enemy, but a life-form containing characteristics of each.

NIH's friendly employees welcomed me, whereas its dreadful food turned me away. So many cancer patients spent their time there. They were Sick Kids, unlike me, even though we shared the same kind of illness and appearance. NIH made them that way, or at least that's how it seemed to me. The hallways and elevators escorted us from one inhuman place to another with the ultimate intention of freeing us from disease, all the while mercilessly punishing us. The machines beeped and buzzed in a foreign language I grew to understand. The rooms, structures, and some of the staff lacked human traits, like empathy, and transposed them onto some of us. That helped me feel, and even be, more like Superman.

NIH helped make me that way by fostering an atmosphere where that feeling could grow, which created a code that I lived by, like "the Code of Harry" in *Dexter*:

- Survive
- Don't cry
- Don't complain
- Don't show pain
- Don't show fear
- Don't question your ability to survive
- Don't question your superiority
- Think of cancer as normal
- Don't let cancer make you sad or jealous

Few other entities were as critical to my growth as that hospital. My faith in the code, like Dexter and his, was shaken, which was the reason I permitted myself to leave NIH. I was so fucked-up that I had to question some of the rules.

Not everyone, including doctors and even Dr. Trout, could become as flawless as the cancer-slaying Super Man that I was at NIH when I had Ewing's. Not even Superman could be Superman all the time. He had to put his time in as Clark Kent. Favorably or not, I will always remember

NIH vividly. Those doctors and nurses are part of the reason I'm alive today, though Dr. Trout I could do without.

Dr. Jennsen's office was closer than NIH, so my checkups took less time. Dr. Jennsen only wanted to see me weekly. She shared my sentiment about my weight. I had fallen from 125 to ninety-eight pounds since leaving for Minnesota, a twenty-two percent drop in body weight. According to the body mass index, I was underweight and approaching severely underweight. Years later, Dr. Jennsen said that she should have photographed me. "You looked like a whole different person," she said.

When I had Ewing's sarcoma, I loved that NIH paid little attention to my nutrition. I felt less pressured. Now, nutrition was the only thing I wanted them to care about. At less than a hundred pounds, I was baffled that no one seemed concerned.

To top it off, I had developed gallstones and couldn't eat fatty foods. I needed a high-calorie, low-fat diet, but I was unable to eat large quantities, which, by my calculations, was impossible. Faced with the prospect of laparoscopic surgery, I listened as my dad said, "You should get your gallbladder removed. While you're asleep, they should also take out your appendix and spleen, because you don't need those things."

"Dad, your spleen is kind of important."

"Are you sure?"

"I think so."

"Then they'll just take your appendix, that's all. I kind of want my gallbladder out. I don't use it," he explained.

With the help of the drug Actigall, some stones turned to sludge and I held off on surgery. Since the stones and sludge never completely disappear, my gallbladder removal is inevitable. Removal of my appendix and spleen, however, is not.

At my six-month post-transplant checkup, I had a lip biopsy, one of the best determinants of GVHD. I had been fearful of graft vs. host disease since my transplant, but by this time I begged for it. My salivary

glands stopped working. I chewed my food until it was mush. Even then I had to gulp water, like I was taking a pill. I tried dry-mouth gum, mouthwash and spray, to no avail. I should have gargled with triamcinolone.

My eyes were dirt dry, which caused excessive tear production. The tears pooled in the bottom of my eyelids until overflowing, first saturating my unnaturally long eyelashes until finally streaming down my cheeks. As a non-crier, I felt the need to prove the salty discharge was not of my accord, like I was guilty until proven innocent.

My lips were so dry I was peeling off thin layers of yellow skin. I slathered myself with moisturizer and steroid creams several times a day. My bowels switched between both extremes. Since GVHD has its own treatment, I figured that would make me healthy again. If it wasn't GVHD, then I didn't know how I would continue surviving.

The following week, I received the phone call from Dr. Fry that I had been anxiously awaiting. "Your lip biopsy showed evidence of GVHD, so you're going to start taking prednisone."

I had never been so happy to have a life-threatening condition. Dr. Fry continued. "Prednisone is a basic steroid. Generally, for chronic GVHD, we have the patient take prednisone as well as cyclosporine. But, since you are almost finished weaning off cyclosporine, you can stop that immediately."

I have a theory on how I developed GVHD. It started during my three-week hospital stay with hemorrhagic cystitis when I stopped eating and moving. The stress I put on my body was enormous. I got a skin biopsy at the end of July, but those aren't accurate determinants for GVHD, and no evidence was found. At NIH, Dr. Bruce began decreasing my dose of cyclosporine, a critical immunosuppressant that helps prevent GVHD from developing. I was weaned off the medication too quickly, which caused symptoms of GVHD to eventually appear. I couldn't wait to begin my steroids. If it didn't work, then traditional ancient Chinese medicine was probably next. Bring on the bear bile and toad venom.

I started at fifty milligrams twice a day, a high dose. Prednisone is hard

on the stomach, causing acid to build up. I had my worst vomit ever during my first evening on prednisone. Acid shot through my nasal cavity, burning my skull. Thick mucus restricted my breathing, and I couldn't blow it out. I rushed to the bathroom and started a hot shower and stuck my face into the steam.

This turned out to be my final transplant-related vomit, and I hadn't even reached a hundred pukes. Over the past months, I had become so used to throwing up that I was nearly addicted to it. I always felt great after a good puke, so if I didn't vomit, I didn't feel right.

The most significant side effect of prednisone is bone thinning. Dr. Jennsen had me get a DEXA scan, which measures bone mineral density. She called with the bad news. "You have osteoporosis."

A voice began screaming inside my head.

"No. That can't be. I'm only nineteen years old."

"You've received so much chemo and radiation that your bones can't produce enough new cells to keep up. There is medication that may reverse the effects and build more bone."

"I just bought a gym membership to get my strength back. What am I supposed to do?"

"You can't lift heavy weight because that can cause a fracture. You have to do very lightweight exercises."

> Date: Tuesday, October 28, 2003
> To: Nick, Terry, Andy, Worm, Drew, Bently
> I found out this morning that I have osteoporosis from all the chemo. Normally I wouldn't complain about shit, but I'm so pissed right now I have to get this off my chest. I always thought that no matter what shit I went through, I would have my strength to bounce back with. I lost all my strength after the bone cancer, and again after the transplant. I just bought a gym membership and planned on getting jacked.

When I wrote that e-mail, my strength had been my shield, my armor. As long as I had my strength, I would get by. Up to this point, I was ready to prove to the world that I had taken on cancer twice, survived each time and still could push my body hard enough to have these shields of muscle. Now, I had the bones of a sixty-year-old woman. Maybe I would never be able to lift heavy weight again.

I had accepted the bone cancer, I had accepted that I had almost no left hip, I had accepted that for the rest of my life I would continuously be rehabbing my hip, and I had even accepted that I would never run or play football again. But now I was having a hard time believing that at nineteen years old, my bones were shot. NIH had never warned me about this and had never given me medication options to prevent this.

At this point, I would have loved to shove a knife into some of the docs. Since I couldn't do that, I thought about punching a hole through a wall. All that would achieve was breaking my hand. Better yet, I could have punched a hole through Dr. Trout and pleaded temporary insanity. After I calmed down, I called Nick. "I know I've asked you this a bunch of times, but I'll ask once more…who's medical history would you rather have?"

"I'll stick with mine," Nick said.

"That's the first time you've said that. I would still rather have mine. I don't want anything to do with AIDS."

"Osteoporosis? I don't want weak bones. Fuck that." Nick was adamant.

While I had been in Minnesota, Nick had developed severe psoriasis, an autoimmune disease of the skin. He too had had his most trying summer, because his psoriasis had turned into erythroderma, a potentially fatal condition in which ninety-eight percent of the skin on his body became red and inflamed. He couldn't regulate his body temperature because all of his blood rose to the surface. Approximately half of people with erythroderma die. In all of his e-mails, Nick hadn't mentioned it, so I hadn't known of his struggle until I got home.

Ever since Nick had told me he had AIDS, I had been asking him if

he would exchange medical conditions with me if he could. He always said yes. Nick's saying no suggested that he thought that recovering my strength might be impossible. I was determined to do it. I obtained a prescription for physical therapy. My former therapist, Kevin Linde, had started his own PT business. This time, he focused on strengthening my entire body instead of just my hip, and he taught me weightlifting exercises that were safe for my fragile bones.

Under Kevin's direction, I lifted weights because I believed a strong body would offset what I was missing elsewhere. I wanted to prove that I was still strong after surviving cancer twice. But the main reason I lifted was because I did not want to be perceived as a weakling. The stronger I appeared, the less likely it was that someone would think of me as a Sick Kid.

When my osteoporosis was later downgraded to osteopenia, I really hit the gym hard. I became obsessed with my body's appearance. Any visual body fat repelled me. I wasn't satisfied until I had the slender body of a Greek god. But, just as cancer treatment zapped my body's ability to create new bone cells, it slowed my muscle generation, as well. I would never look like Ares.

I'm still not secure with my appearance. I was never tall, strong, lean or tan enough. My teeth were never straight or white enough. I had too many freckles. I believed that the correction of a physical characteristic would have a similar attractive effect on my personality. I wasn't self-confident when Andrea wrote her phone number in my yearbook, hoping I would ask her out. Imagine how I felt when I could no longer hide under the mop of hair on my head. On Halloween, even though I was nineteen, I dressed up like a kid. I covered up all evidence of my cancer with a badass Undertaker mask.

Birdsall and I went trick-or-treating. Some thought we were too old, but we wanted our candy. I walked around with my Undertaker mask while he sported sunglasses and a raincoat, claiming to be Neo from *The Matrix*. When we approached the neighbors' houses, they would be ready

to distribute handfuls of sweets. But when they saw that I was nineteen and Birdsall was twenty, they grabbed one piece for each of us, not realizing that adults need more calories than children. Little did I know then that this Halloween would be the last time I could eat commercial candies. After nearly two decades of sugar consumption, I began to develop allergies I had never had before from the transplant.

My first allergic reaction occurred several hours after receiving pamidronate, a drug used to prevent bone breakdown and fractures. I started to itch. Hives broke out all over my body, and my tongue swelled. I took Benadryl and went to the ER. On the way, my throat closed, and my chest tightened. I was afraid of not being able to breathe. The Benadryl reversed the reaction soon after I got to the ER.

Over the coming months, I had countless severe reactions—once after eating a Tastykake, and another time because of Rollos. I was crushed when I finally discovered that milk was causing my allergic reactions, and that I would never drink Fuddruckers strawberry milkshakes again. I switched to grape juice with my meals, but I kept spilling on my shirt and staining my clothes. As a last resort, I turned to my old friend, water. Do you know what water tastes like? It tastes like nothing.

Jonathan said, "If you're allergic to pizza, then you'll just have to take Benadryl and hope for the best." Thankfully I didn't react to most cooked cheeses and continued eating pizza without having to jab myself with an EpiPen.

My old allergist tested me and results showed that I was at least mildly allergic to forty-three items, including twenty-five foods and seven animals. Is that it? "Stay away from the cow," he told me. But according to my new allergist, nobody has ever been documented to have more than a few food allergies. My allergies may have come from my bone marrow donor, but no hard feelings. I still love her.

When every organ seemed to be deteriorating, and every muscle at-

rophying, and my life slipping away, I became well. The cure wasn't oxycodone or Valium, or an experimental treatment, or an invasive procedure, but the simple steroid, prednisone, which gave back my life force.

Sixteen-year-old Ben would have recovered after his transplant months before nineteen-year-old Ben did. It would seem that his inner Super Man was dead and gone, leaving simple Ben, capeless. That thought was as pitiful to me as my appearance.

I hadn't used the term Super Man as a joke. It was my strengths in fighting cancer that led me to believe I was a Super Man. No other term could describe my extraordinary resilience to disease and my capacity to survive the cure. Obstacles were thrown up to me constantly and I resisted them because of my super powers. Super describes what was extraordinary about me but maybe the superhuman Ben was an inhuman Ben. Unlike my cancer-ridden left ilium, my Super Man complex was the one thing I had that no one could take away. Like the code I continue to uphold, my faith in my super powers remained. My invisible cape is still tied around my neck. No matter how it seems I should feel about these amazing powers, they will always be a part of me, even if they are nothing other but a remnant, like a single cancer cell that can't be killed, waiting for its time to flourish again.

All my problems disappeared almost instantly. Birdsall immediately noticed my uplifted spirits. While throwing the Nerf football with me, he said, "The steroids seem to be working, huh?"

"Yeah, it's awesome."

"Before you looked lifeless, and now you're rifling this ball at me. I'm afraid if I piss you off you'll get 'roid rage.'"

"Dude, you're thinking of anabolic steroids."

I had so much energy you'd think I was on speed. My constant state of euphoria only supplemented it. I had trouble sleeping because my mind would race. I would have multiple thoughts streaming through my brain, unable to control them. Sometimes I would prop my head and

shoulders up with pillows and visualize lying on the retractable bed in Room 210 in Minnesota. I would listen for the rumbling of the HEPA filter in the ceiling which now seemed soothing in an odd way. That combination often put me to sleep. I still do the pillow trick but have forgotten what the HEPA filter sounded like. I think that's a good thing.

The only benefit to losing twenty-seven pounds was regaining it. I ate four meals a day and was always hungry for snacks. Everything was delicious, and I devoured it all, without discriminating against nutritious vegetables. My daily caloric intake shot from around 1,300 to several thousand.

My primary short-term goal had been to acquire an appetite by Thanksgiving. I succeeded, starving myself all day and gorging myself at dinner with my mom's turkey, cranberry sauce, and famous stuffing.

I knew I would fully recover while at T.G.I. Friday's with Jonathan, a few days after I started prednisone. I ordered the bacon cheeseburger and fries, assuming I would take most of it home. When I cleaned my plate, I bragged to Jonathan about it for the rest of the day.

Sundays were heavenly. Jonathan, my dad and I ordered NFL Sunday Ticket, which allowed us to choose which games we wanted to watch. Unless the house was burning down, you could not have moved me from my fifty-three-inch sweetheart. When the Redskins played, we were tempted to switch to a different game, but couldn't bring ourselves to do it. They had a dismal 2003 season, going 5-11.

For lunch each Sunday, Jonathan and I ordered pizza. It's a continuing tradition I call The Sunday Special. Nick once asked me what made it special. "Do you get it from somewhere specific? Is there a special deal or a special kind of pizza you always get?"

"No. Any pizza from anywhere at any price."

"But that's not a special. You have to change the name."

"It's special to me, so back off."

I spent time with Jonathan every chance I got. Most of my friends were away at college, and Jonathan was working part-time at Domino's

and was home often. We watched the first two seasons of *24* on DVD in the span of five days. We joked that we should have watched each season straight through without breaks. "It'll only be about seventeen hours," we said. We went to lunch and saw a movie in the theaters each week. He even took me to most of my checkups. I don't know if he enjoyed our time together, but I found it rewarding.

Jonathan could have lived with friends in Arlington, but he stayed home to be with me. In November, he received another offer to move in with friends, but declined because I wasn't sure whether or not I would be back to school the following semester. When I finally decided to return to UVA early in December, he lost his opportunity to move out and stayed at home until the end of the summer. Jonathan rearranged his whole life for me for over a year.

During the first three months after prednisone restored my life, I was content with precisely what I had. I may not have been rich, famous, or had the hottest girlfriend (or any girlfriend), but screw it. There was nothing more that I desired. Everything felt special, from going to my weekly checkups with Jonathan, to watching the 6:00 p.m. edition of *SportsCenter*. This may sound boring and ordinary, but for me it was Utopia. I had never been happier over a stretch of time that long. Once again, I would give my big left nut to experience it again.

One thing wasn't perfect though: my friends were moving on. At winter break, when they came home from school, I saw it clearly again. I felt like a stranger at Drew's house when we played poker—the first time I'd seen them in a year. Drew's house had always been a second home to me. We used to decide whose house we'd hang out at by flipping a pillow—smooth side my house, rough side his. I went to his house every Christmas to play with his gifts and join them for Christmas dinner. I used to eat dinner at his house as often as possible because his dad was such a good cook. We created new sports in our basements, such as a putt-putt course or *American Gladiators* with Nerf guns. During the blizzard of '96, I slept

at his house three nights in a row. I used to enter so informally that his dad called me Cosmo Kramer after the neighbor in *Seinfeld*.

Why did everything have to change just because I had had a transplant? Why did cancer have to cut me out of so much? But, my friends, as reliable with their jokes as ever before, used their skills to make me feel welcome and lightened the mood when things got awkward. They made fun of the food at Don Pablo's, of Andy's waiting skills and of Worm for being Worm. They treated me like I was the same Ben and made Drew's house feel like home, again. But I knew in a few weeks they would go back to their new lives and I would restart mine after a year-long hiatus. I wanted to get back to school but even more I wanted to get back to normal.

It was a great moment when my Hickman catheter was removed. I could move on. I returned to the University of Virginia and lived with three high school friends, including Tim Castellar, who would remain my roommate for the duration of college. After getting busted for alcohol by his parents, Tim's mom started calling him, "My Little Alky." He'd been drinking since middle school. Tim may have been a drunk but he was a sharp mind and a good friend.

Back in our senior year of high school, before we became close friends, Tim initiated conversation about my cancer experiences. Bently was shocked, and thought I would be offended. Instead, I was impressed that Tim asked questions that many lacked the courage to ask.

I didn't invite Derek to live with us. Even after my second cancer and despite Derek's staunch devotion to me, I still didn't understand that new friends could become equal to old ones, though Derek and I still met often for drinking or sporting events. At the end of January, as I was riding in the car with Tim, my mom called. "Benjamin, I'm at the hospital with Dad. This was the first chance I had to call you."

"Why? What happened?" My stomach churned, as if I had eaten salmon.

"Dad slipped on the ice walking up the driveway, and broke his wrist."

Relief swept over me. "Is that it? Is he okay?"

"He'll be fine. The doctors have him doped up so he's sleeping in a chair right now."

"Are they going to fix his arm?"

"Yes, after they look at the X-rays."

"Okay. He needs to be more careful, you know?"

"Yes, he does. Benjamin, I think you should know something."

"What is it?"

"After he slipped, he rushed into my office and he was crying."

"Dad was crying?"

"He was terrified, and kept saying that he can't help you any more and he doesn't know what to do."

"What are you talking about? I don't need any help."

"I think he was just shocked. I could see the bone out of place under the skin."

"Wait, wait. What did he mean? Why was he crying about me?"

"He said that he won't be able to help you pack your computer and other things when you come home for the summer. He was all out of sorts until they gave him a sedative. But I don't want you to worry. I'll call you later." Tim stared at me waiting for an explanation, but I kept silent. I said maybe ten words the rest of the evening.

I knew my cancers affected my parents differently. I fear that all the trauma permanently scarred my mom's brain, and she would never be the same. I think my mom felt responsible for my cancer, like she had eaten the wrong foods during pregnancy. She probably blamed herself for not noticing my pain after tennis practice when I was sixteen and getting me to the doctor sooner.

It was less obvious to me that my dad struggled with my cancers too. I noticed a couple of little things, but I thought that they were just part of being a father to a Sick Kid: Always a man of unchanging habits, he adjusted his quirks, like avoiding travel, for me. Always someone who denied emotion, he consulted the social worker, Ronne

at NIH, to understand how to help me better. Dad must have felt that when he broke his wrist, his ability to assist me was compromised. He actually broke down and cried because of that. I was shocked. I had thought that, unlike my mom's, his suffering because of my illness was fairly superficial.

I continued to push my parents away, and stopped answering when they asked how I was feeling. I avoided saying anything negative around them. I kept my feelings to myself. But no matter what I did to detach them from me, nothing drove them away. Eventually, I came to understand the value of a support team. I used to mock patients for even mouthing the word "support," but if it hadn't been for my family, my faith in my recovery might have been shattered.

When the body has endured so much, the patient tends to notice things about it all the time. I woke up hungover after celebrating my bone marrow's first birthday. I stepped out of bed and felt a jagged pain deep inside my left hip. After stretching, I took another step and felt the same sting. Did I sleep in a funny position? Did I hurt myself at the gym yesterday?

At some point in my life, I had been accustomed to this exact same pain, but I couldn't pinpoint it this time. I never expected to use my crutches again, so I had left them at my parents' house. I would grab a pair at Student Health when it opened the next day. So, I popped a few oxycodones and watched movies all day.

For three straight days, the sharp pain persisted. If it was a strained muscle, then it should have gone away by now. I doubted that I had dislocated something. Maybe one of the staples tore through the muscle. Maybe…no, it can't be…cancer?

The last time I felt this pain was back when I was playing tennis during my sophomore year of high school. I phoned Dr. Jennsen.

"Do you think the Ewing's is back?" I asked her.

"No. Cancer wouldn't have caused such an acute pain after you woke up."

"Maybe your hip joint collapsed," she suggested.

"Am I going to need surgery?"

"I don't know," she said. "We'll need to get you in for scans."

I headed to Nick's apartment to talk to him and Terry. "It started again. I have a sharp pain in my hip. I think it might be cancer again. Looks like I'm going for Round III."

"You don't know that yet," Nick said.

"My doctor doesn't think its cancer, but I can't stop considering the possibility."

"What else could it be?" Terry asked.

"My hip joint might be completely destroyed. I may need surgery and have to rehab all over again. I don't know if I can handle that shit again. I was doing so well, too. It's just not fair."

One week later, I received hip and chest CT scans. I was terrified that I had cancer, but I had to know.

I held my breath when Dr. Jennsen entered my room.

"No cancer!" she said.

"Are you sure?"

"Yes. You're perfectly healthy."

"Wow. Thank you so much. So I don't need surgery?"

"Absolutely not. Sorry your summer started off like this, but things look good."

Five days later, I was with Dr. Wodajo, discussing my scan results. "Your joint looks like it did last year," he said.

"Then what caused the sharp pain?" I asked.

"It's hard to say. Is it gone now?"

"I don't know. I've been using crutches and haven't tested it."

"Take some laps in the hall to see if you feel any pain."

I hopped off the examination table, crutched my way out to the hall, and leaned the crutches against the wall. I carefully took a couple of steps and stopped. "I think it's gone!"

I took some pain-free laps in the hallway.

"What happened? Why did it just disappear?" I asked him.

"There's no way to know, but it's possible that a thin piece of tissue found its way into your hip joint, causing the pain, and then worked itself out." When I got home later that afternoon, I shoved my crutches back into the closet where they belonged.

Just after returning to school following summer break, I saw green diarrhea after my morning dump. I went to class assuming I contracted a gut virus, but when I got back home, my stomach was red and itchy. I called Dr. Jennsen's office. "You need to get that biopsied," the nurse said, after I described to her my symptoms. "Call back later and tell me what happened. If I'm not here, leave a message."

I hadn't been to UVA Medical Center in about a year-and-a-half, and she expected me to get a dermatology appointment on the spot? I called the Hematology/Oncology clinic where I used to go for platelet transfusions.

"Hi, I'm Ben Rubenstein, I used to be a patient here. May I speak to the doctor I used to see? Maybe his name starts with a P?"

I could just as easily have been speaking to her in Xhosa, so I grabbed my car keys. I would take care of this my way. I steered with one hand and scratched with the other until I got to UVA Medical Center. When I reached the front desk at the Dermatology clinic, I said, "My skin is having problems, is there something you can do for me?"

"No, you'd have to obtain a referral to see us."

By this time, the itching was so unbearable that I thought I might shred my skin. I took the elevator to where the Pediatric Hematology/ Oncology clinic used to be. "I used to come here. Is this the Hematology clinic?"

"No, you need to go over there," the woman at the desk said and pointed to the left.

I started walking away when another nurse spotted me. "Ben, is that you?"

I turned to see the short nurse with the brown hair and brown eyes,

one of so many who have cared for me over the years, and had no recollection of her name. "Uh yeah."

"How are you, it's been a while, huh?"

"Yeah, I guess it has. Does doctor…I can't remember his name…?"

"Dr. Peters?" she asked.

"Yes, that's it! Does he still work here? My skin is going nuts, and I cannot stop scratching."

"He sure does. Let me see if we can fit you in this afternoon."

I paced around as patients peered at me like I was crazy. I kept rubbing water on my stomach, which provided brief, yet amazing, relief. I'll take pain over this itching any day.

The nurse who recognized me sneaked me in to see Dr. Peters, who examined my skin.

"That doesn't look like GVHD, but I can't be certain. We'll schedule you for a biopsy over at Dermatology. In the meantime, let me give you IV Benadryl to hopefully relieve your itch."

My skin biopsy the following week didn't exhibit GVHD. "You have a bad case of eczema, or dry skin," the dermatologist said.

For the next two years, I went through Eucerin, steroid cream and Benadryl like Jonathan goes through Starbursts. My Benadryl count must have been over 1,000. My sleep was often disrupted because of the scratching. For many people, eczema only develops on certain parts of their body, like the face or arms. My eczema, however, showed its ugly face anywhere and everywhere, any day and every day. My allergist explained the link between eczema and allergies, and I now keep my eczema under control with allergy shots.

My diarrhea showed a similar tenacity. Although my green poop eventually disappeared, my diarrhea didn't. Colostomy bag continued to haunt me. Dr. Jennsen wanted to check for viruses in my stool when I saw her for a checkup. I was supposed to poop in a bucket, and then scoop it into two vials, but I only filled one of them. So, I went back

into the bathroom, grabbed the bucket out of the trashcan, scraped the excess shit that I hadn't flushed down the toilet, and dropped it into the second vial. It still wasn't enough, so I drove to Wendy's across the street thinking a spicy chicken sandwich and loaded baked potato would get me shitting. I came back and tried to crap, without success. Dr. Jennsen sent me home and said not to worry about it. The results were negative for infection, anyway.

Several weeks later, I had a colonoscopy.

"You don't have GVHD," the gastroenterologist said. "Your diarrhea is caused by irritable bowel syndrome."

In the summer of 2005, I met with a radiation oncologist at NIH. "Do you think my irritable bowel syndrome is caused by radiation?" I asked him.

"Yes."

"But my CT scan looks normal, and the colonoscopy was normal."

"I think that the radiation caused small blood vessel disease in your intestines so it's no surprise that everything looks normal. It should improve over time."

"You don't think I'll need surgery in the future, do you? Because before I had total body irradiation, the doctor had said I may need surgery and possibly a colostomy bag."

"No, I wouldn't worry about that."

Fortunately, my irritable bowel syndrome improved.

Again, following summer break, I had another incident at school. "I have a bruise on my leg," I said to my roommate, Tim, after looking down at my shin.

"Maybe you bumped it."

"Maybe. But the last time this happened, it was myelodysplasia."

Once I considered the tinniest possibility that I had cancer, my rational thinking went haywire. Even if I tried relaxing and telling myself that it was nothing, the cancer ghosts would intervene. What if it turned out to be something? What if it was a precursor to something grave?

"What do you wanna do?" Tim asked.

"I won't sleep until I find out if my myelodysplasia is back. I have to get a blood test, but Student Health is closed."

"You want me to drive you to the ER?"

"No, that'd be crazy. I don't think they'd even take me seriously. I'll just go to Student Health first thing in the morning."

Tim left the room, so I tried focusing on my macroeconomics book, but I kept reading the same sentence without realizing it. I set the book down and thought about whether I had recently bumped my leg.

Tim returned and said, "I just talked with somebody at the ER. She said they'd be more than happy doing a blood test tonight."

Once there, we waited almost two hours before my blood was taken, as Tim performed tricks on a wheelchair that was lying around. Then a doctor entered and said, "Great news. Your platelets are 230 thousand."

Everything was normal. I must have bumped my leg, but several months later, I noticed a change in my hip. My range of motion, which was once great for a nearly free-floating hip joint, became severely limited. Leg lifts, which I used to perform with such ease, became painful. Raising my leg into my car became impossible without assisting with my arm. Anytime I stood from a seated position, I would stretch before walking, which was still painful for the first few steps. I even lost the ability to ride a bike.

"Your hip joint is destroyed," Dr. Merlin said when I met with him about it.

"What do you mean? Is the X-ray worse than last year's?"

"Yes. The end of your femur and socket are completely dead. Your pain is from inflammation in your hip caused by the bones rubbing together. Actually, you don't even have a joint anymore."

"What will happen in the future? Is it going to worsen? Will I need hip replacement surgery?"

"We could do that if you had a hip, but you don't have anything to

replace. You don't have any bone there. If your pain gets worse, we may be able to surgically fuse your femur to your pelvis."

"Wouldn't I be walking around like Frankenstein?"

"Your limp would be magnified, but it would help ease your pain."

After a long pause, I said, "This is pretty disappointing."

"Well, at least you don't have cancer or infection."

"Yeah, I guess."

"Stay off your leg for two weeks, and take it easy for another six weeks."

"Do I have to go back on crutches?"

"Yes. There's too much inflammation in there. After two weeks, you can stop using crutches, but you need to limit your walking and movement for another six weeks."

"You mean that you want me to stop doing my hip exercises?"

"For now."

A slideshow of memories of Dr. Merlin praising me ran through my head on the ride home. I couldn't believe how he had shifted on me, telling me now so nonchalantly that the future of my hip was downhill. How can I do that after dedicating the last five years of my life to strengthening my hip? Now he was telling me exercising was a waste? I did every thing he asked me to do, and now I'm supposed to sit back and watch my hip vaporize?

So, about a month later, I saw Dr. Wodajo for a second opinion. "From the new X-ray, you can see that your hip has experienced extensive damage since the last X-ray," he said.

I looked at the front view of my pelvis and gasped. The picture was incredibly different from the X-ray taken six months after my surgery, in which all the bones were clearly defined. I couldn't even tell where my femur joined my hip socket. There was a cluster of body parts.

"As you can see, the radiation deformed the bones, so now your hip joint has become much flatter due to a collapse of the weight-bearing dome. Your femoral head has also flattened. Your hip joint has tilted more, causing the

femoral head to shift further up the joint, closer to your abdomen."

"Is that why I feel a bigger dip in my steps?"

"Yes. You may need a bigger lift in that left shoe."

"So how much worse is it going to get?"

"The only way to know is for you to get a CT scan."

"Let's say it does get worse. Is surgery a possibility? Dr. Merlin had mentioned a surgery where the femur can be fused to the hip."

"We have three options. The fusing surgery is the first, but that would really limit your mobility. The second option is to surgically place some fresh bone on top of your hip joint in order to stop it from migrating up. I don't want to do that either, because your blood flow in that area is poor. The bone may not even survive. The third option is to do nothing. You need to try to save your hip for as long as possible. If you save what's left of it, then it may not get much worse. I think you should start using a cane. Also, limit your walking. Don't go on any long hikes."

"A cane? For how long?"

"Forever."

"I can't do that."

"Why not?"

"I can't go back to that. It would be a huge leap backwards. If I have to use something, then I would much prefer to use a crutch. I know it sounds stupid, but people treat you differently with a cane."

"Okay."

"This really sucks."

"I know it does," he said.

"Did you know this was eventually going to happen?"

"It was bound to happen because you don't have anything there to stop it. Frankly, I'm surprised this didn't happen sooner. So, get your CT scan and come back in two weeks."

I had too much pride. I met Bently at a bar and told him what Dr. Wodajo said. "Where's your cane?" Bently asked.

"Forget that. First of all, he doesn't know if it's necessary. He has to look at the CT scan, first."

"Damn it, Ben, don't be an idiot."

"If he looks at the CT scan and tells me I need to use a cane, then I may consider it."

"You better use it. It's your future, man. Don't worry about what other people think. You do what you have to do."

"That's easier said than done. You have no idea how hard that would be."

When I got home, I went down to the closet, and grabbed my cane. The grip was soft and torn. "Suck it up and do it," I urged myself. I began leaning on the cane as I headed upstairs to my bedroom. For the next two weeks, I used the cane at home, but I couldn't use it in public. I desperately hoped the CT scan would show something different. When I saw Dr. Wodajo, it did.

"This looks much better than I originally thought," Dr. Wodajo said, after looking at the CT scans. "Your femur's force looks equally distributed between your hip and scar tissue. Scar tissue is tough, so I don't think your femur will move much more. The bone-on-bone contact is what's causing your pain. In fact, if your femur does slip further up your joint, I think it may actually relieve some of your pain."

"What about the cane?"

"Forget about that. I don't think you can damage it much further. I'm not saying you should go run a marathon, but you certainly don't need to walk around with a cane."

"You have no idea how happy that makes me to hear you say that. You're the man, Dr. Wodajo."

Toward the end of the summer, I had two physical therapy sessions with Kevin, and he taught me exercises to improve my strength. That, combined with a larger lift in my shoe, decreased my pain. I still experienced some pain, but it didn't bother me because I became used to it.

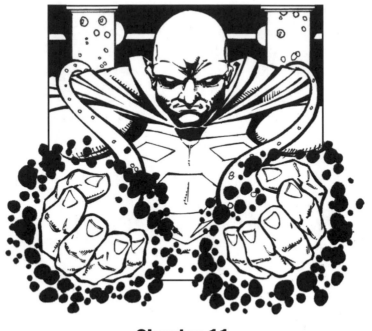

Chapter 11
FIGHTING THE FEAR

Over the course of my life, it is likely my wonder hip will further deteriorate. My continued health has provided me the opportunity to look towards the future, something I couldn't do with cancer. I have taken Dr. Wodajo's original advice and focused on saving my hip. I may not ever run or play football again, but I can walk slowly with the best of them.

With my hip taken care of, I began to focus on the rest of my body. I got a MUGA scan as part of my five-year restaging. This test produces the ejection fraction of the heart, or in other words, the percent of blood the left ventricle pumps with each beat. A normal ejection fraction is at least fifty-five percent.

"The preliminary results show forty-five percent," Christine said.

An eerie sensation overcame me and I felt that I was back in her old

office after she had just told me my platelets were 24 thousand. Christine saw that I was distraught and said, "What's the problem?"

"What was my MUGA result the last time, because I don't remember it ever being this low?"

She looked through my chart in search of a normally meaningless number. "The last time you got a MUGA was two years ago, and it was fifty-seven."

"I dropped twelve points in just two years?"

"Your preliminary results came from a tech, and I know this guy; he often is off by as many as ten points. This doesn't mean anything."

"Did the Adriamycin cause this?"

"It might have."

"If forty-five percent is accurate, and the Adriamycin damaged my heart, is there any way to prevent more damage?"

"No, but there is medication that can help with the symptoms. I know people who have ejection fractions in the thirties, but they're doing just fine. I wouldn't expect your ejection fraction to drop any more. Ben, we're getting ahead of ourselves. Let's wait for the official results and then talk about it."

When I got home, I googled heart damage resulting from Adriamycin. What I found made my skin crawl. What had my total dose been? Did I surpass my lifetime limit? Had I developed cardiotoxicity? Was my heart going to fail? Was I going to need a heart transplant? Was I going to need a pacemaker? How the hell was I supposed to tell my parents that their youngest son's heart was failing?

Christine called with the results at the end of the week.

"The tech was right, the number is forty-five percent," she said.

I started shaking. "Does that mean I'm going to have heart failure?"

"Of course not. It's just a number. These things vary. There are countless reasons why yours was low, and if you had another MUGA, I bet it would be higher. Really, Ben, don't worry about this. You're going to be just fine."

One week later, I had an echocardiogram which showed a left ventricle ejection fraction of fifty-six percent, eleven percent higher than the MUGA. Two months later, a stress test showed my heart was completely normal—no blockages, no arrhythmias, normal function, sixty-five percent ejection fraction, and eighty-nine percent normal reaction to stress. Three years later an echocardiogram showed a drop, an ejection fraction of forty-five percent and then a significant increase a year later to seventy-four percent. I will always have a risk of developing cardiotoxicity resulting from the Adriamycin doses I had received, assuming it hasn't already happened. It is said that the human heart has a maximum number of ticks.

Tick-tock. Tick-tock.

A long time ago, when I was a little kid, I was scared of thunderstorms. During late night storms, I would sleep on Jonathan's floor in my sleeping bag. In the morning when my dad woke him up for school, I would sleepwalk back to my room.

My silly fears didn't end with thunderstorms. Fireworks, ailens, robbers, and certain "heel" wrestlers also gave me the creeps. Those fears might have faded, but they were superseded by something much worse: every change my body goes through I attribute to something disastrous. In a way, I have become what my mom has always been. Maybe I am a little bit crazy. Maybe this is a natural process the mind goes through for protection. All I know is that unless I can force The Fear to wear my Super-Jew shirt, it will stay with me forever.

I have been cancer-free from both diseases for over seven years. I could call myself cured, although I don't. My risk of developing cancer is about as low as it will ever be again. I'm also as healthy and physically strong as I have been in years. But a first-rate immune system and less than ten percent body fat do not protect me from cancer. That's what my organic Gala apples are for.

When my hemoglobin still had not fully recovered two years after

my transplant, Dr. Jennsen performed a blood test and found that I have a thalassemia trait. That's a genetic blood disorder that often occurs in people of Mediterranean descent, which is likely the ethnicity of my donor. Normal hemoglobin is composed of four proteins, and one of mine doesn't function properly. My new bone marrow still produces the normal amount of red blood cells, they're just smaller.

For the rest of my life I will be anemic, and my heart rate increases with little physical exertion. I am more interested in strengthening my heart, and hoping that my heart is racing because of anemia and not cardiotoxicity.

After every checkup Bently always asked, "You got a clean bill of health, right?"

My bill of health isn't the same as most. After my transplant I developed a phosphorus deficiency. Dr. Jennsen said my kidneys excrete too much of the mineral. When I asked if the condition would worsen, she said no. I thought about how shitty it was for a minute and then moved on. It won't get worse, there's nothing I can do about it, and I'm perfectly capable of taking phosphorus supplements, so what's the problem?

My chances of developing serious health problems, such as cancer or organ dysfunction, are astronomically higher than normal. I'm one of the millions of cancer survivors—literally millions—striving to live a normal, healthy life in this crazy, mixed-up world. In 2007, I graduated with a degree in economics from the University of Virginia. Maybe I will find myself a pretty young lady to marry and utilize my frozen sperm. Who knows?

I would be greedy if I complained about nuisances, as doctors continue to describe my non life-threatening disorders. If a single aspect of my transplant had been changed, it could have triggered the butterfly effect. Then maybe I would be dead.

My donor may know who she is if she is reading this. She was born in New York in 1999, likely of Mediterranean descent, possesses

thalassemia, has the blood type O+, possibly has allergies and dry skin, and her mother had donated her umbilical cord. I want to go on record and thank my donor and her mother for giving me life.

One night in early 2005, Worm, Drew and his new girlfriend, Aubrey Sloane, visited UVA for Terry's twenty-first birthday party. While waiting to return to the beer pong table, Drew asked if this was the first time I had met Aubrey.

"Yeah, I guess it is," I slurred.

"I've heard a lot about you," she said. "Drew refers to you as Benjy."

"Oh yeah? That's funny."

"Ben's my homie," Drew said to her. "We've been best friends our whole lives."

"It's true, we've known each other since we were babies," I said to Aubrey. "Dude, I'm glad to hear you say that. For a while it seemed like we were drifting apart. You know, with the whole cancer thing, then going to different colleges, then the other cancer thing."

"No way. It's always been you, me, Worm and Andy. It'll always be that way."

To me, that drunken conversation was priceless. I thought of the infinite amount of time we had spent together, all the games we played as kids, our hilarious conversations that only we understood and the goofy things we had done together.

After graduating, Nick and Terry remained in Charlottesville and got married. Terry works as a nurse at UVA Medical Center. Some others also stayed in Virginia: Tim in Virginia Beach, Birdsall in Harrisonburg, Worm in Arlington and Rick in Richmond. Derek completed a Ph.D. program in Williamsburg. Friedman and Bently fled to California and lost contact with just about everyone. Andy landed a job in Charlotte and Drew followed soon after.

I used to feel like they all abandoned me, but the reality is that

they moved on with their lives. They developed close friendships with other people. Their lives flowed the way a river meanders and carves new bends, whereas I damned my river, trying to keep everything the same as when I was sixteen.

My loyalty to these friends, as well as to Pre-Cancer Ben, will endure. But in terms of closeness, Nick is unrivaled. Our deadly diseases have connected us. There are only a few drugs left to attack Nick's mutated virus because he has already tried most of them. The last time Worm and I visited Nick in the hospital we never expected to see him again. He had been running a fever for weeks, and when his temperature reached 105, he requested a priest to administer his last rites. As he sat on the side of the bed slipping into the darkness, Terry sat on the opposite side, silencing her mighty sobs so Nick didn't have to hear. Nick survived, like he and I always do, and was placed on a new AIDS cocktail and has seen his viral load drop from over a million to undetectable. The new drugs are his miracle juice.

Nick had always been willing to consider his death. When he nearly died, I felt like a large hole would soon open inside of me that would never be filled. His death would devastate me, and selfishly I contemplated how nobody knows me like he does. It would take years to build a friendship like we already had. If I was ever going to move past sixteen, then maybe I should start reaching out to people the way Nick does.

Toward the end of 2005, while driving him home, Bently said, "Benjy, I'm disappointed in you."

"Disappointed? That's harsh."

"No, not disappointed. I'm just worried about you. You have to get your feet wet, man. I feel like you're not living life to the fullest."

After I dropped him off, his comment lingered. It hadn't been more than an hour since I watched him snort lines of painkiller, smoke a pack of cigarettes, and drink five beers and a 40, and I couldn't help but think, "Maybe I'm not living life to the fullest. Maybe I'm not doing everything that a

college student should be doing. Maybe I'm less of a risk-taker because of cancer. It took away my hip, and maybe I consider the effects it has on my liver, heart, and kidneys, and decide that risks just aren't for me."

Sometimes I wonder if cancer has given me an extra purpose, like I'm supposed to create something spectacular. Maybe all I ever wanted was to be normal. Are expectations higher or lower for survivors? Am I held to higher morals, yet lower accomplishment standards? Why does everyone expect so much of me? Why do I expect so much of myself?

I used to have an amazing ability to manufacture an adrenaline rush and transform my sadness into anger, and then anger into motivation. Anger became my outlet, but I wasn't angry all the time. Actually, I was the opposite. I accepted cancer as a routine. It was when deep sadness opened the door that I became angry. I had an intense fear of vulnerability. I thought depression was hocus-pocus, and even considered those who suffered from it inferior. I realized that I had short stints of sadness, but always recovered quickly. People who suffered from chronic depression disgusted me.

My viewpoint changed after Dr. Wodajo said my hip was fine, when tissue found its way into my joint and worked itself out. I had expected my happiness to return. Two weeks later, my mom and I walked down the clean streets of Minneapolis after my one-year, post-transplant checkup. We passed by the campus, and our old apartment building where my dad needed thirteen three-point turns to park the Big Red Box in the garage, and Leaning Tower of Pizza where I ate my final supper before sixty-five consecutive days in the hospital. But, I was still sad. With the cancer behind me, I could finally confront what had happened to me. I had heard from the docs and social workers that many cancer survivors get depressed about it long after they finish treatment.

I'm still fairly content. Nowadays, whenever I'm feeling down, I give myself pep talks. "You survived cancer twice, what are you so sad about? Man the fuck up." If this doesn't work, I mentally place myself back in

my germfree hospital room with the huge window and think, "Look how far you've come. You should just be happy to be alive."

I need to learn how to address those feelings instead of putting them off. Nevertheless, my method always works. It just takes longer than it used to. I'm not very religious. I go to temple maybe three times a year, but my dad attends services every Friday night. It is traditional in our congregation to sing "Mi Shebeirach," a song about healing. The words go:

> May the source of strength who blessed the ones before us,
> Help us find the courage to make our lives a blessing.
> Bless those in need of healing with refuah sh'leimah
> The renewal of body, the renewal of spirit.

Before singing, the rabbi reads a list naming people who are ill and in need of strength. For years, my name was listed and I couldn't stand it. Sometimes, congregates would ask, "Ben, how are you doing? Are you okay?" as if my funeral were quickly approaching. Someone had the nerve to question me that same way over four years after my transplant. I politely responded that I was fantastic, about to graduate, healthy as an ox and strong as a bull. I wanted to break her neck.

Before Yom Kippur services in 2004, I approached our rabbi and said, "Could you please take me off the "Mi Shebeirach" list? I've been healthy for some time now. My dad will tell you I need to be on the list, but don't listen to him."

The rabbi honored my plea and stopped naming me. That didn't prevent my dad from raising his hand and calling out my name, anyway. I finally yelled at him, and he claims to have stopped except, of course, when I have the sniffles or a paper cut.

My father had been just as protective of me as my mother had but it wasn't until after cancer that I recognized this. Then, when I performed physical activity, like shoveling snow, my dad would say, "No, you stay inside. You don't need to be doing that." This angered me, and of course I would shovel faster and harder.

In ninth grade I had taken over mowing duties from my dad. I became a great mower, and my dad referred to me as a professional. Then when I got cancer, I stopped mowing and it was my dad's responsibility again. I theorized that if I could show him I was fine, then eventually he would believe it. I tested this theory when I tried to take back the mowing duties from my dad.

"I could help you with mowing the grass," I suggested to him.

"Oh no," my dad said. "I can take care of it."

Just like old times I got angry. "It is only cutting the grass. It's not like I am mowing down rows of ragweed which would set off an allergic reaction worth fifty Tastykakes."

"I'm glad of your help, Benjy," he said. Then he paused before he turned off the lawn mower: "Are you sure you feel up to it?" From then on I made a point of doing the mowing while my dad was at work. At first I thought that he didn't notice that I was taking care of the lawn the way I used to. Then one day he called me a professional mower again. It was like he had forgotten that there was ever a time when I hadn't mowed. In a way, because he was such a creature of habit it was easier for me to get back to normal with my dad than it was with my mom.

I was born highly capable of dealing with cancer, the same way Kobe Bryant was born highly capable of playing basketball. Aside from my shot, I'm not very good at basketball, and maybe Kobe wouldn't be very good at fighting cancer. In my opinion, he's the best basketball player in the world. Through a combination of inherent and learned factors, maybe I was the Greatest Cancer Patient Ever. Does that make me a Super Man? Now that I am away from cancer and can relax a little, I wonder.

My personality type made me less prone to complaining. I was able to keep the cancer from bringing me down. Just as I had pushed away my family and friends, I shrugged off the hideous, unpleasant things that happened to me. It didn't matter what was going on around me, whether it was good or bad. I endured cancer the way I played tennis: I was a

pusher. So long as I could run to the ball, I always had a chance to win.

The conviction that I had super powers came to me all at once. It was not logical like my assessment of my body's healing ability. I blindly believed in these powers. I simply created an Ideal Ben and forced myself to live up to the standards of a Super Man. The rules were that if I began to feel sad, jealous, angry or whiny, then I would immediately shut down. It reached a point where if I was supposed to feel something, I suspended my reaction. And if I got bummed out, I immediately turned off my emotions. I sometimes heard people talk about waking up sad, but I couldn't relate to that. My will was so strong, my self-control so great, that this never happened to me.

Other people acted the way human beings were supposed to, but I was certain I didn't need to be a person. I felt extremely unique, and this feeling was amazing and addictive. That uniqueness became the energy source of my super powers.

A shrink would say I didn't have to decide between retaining that feeling of uniqueness and still being emotionally open to others. It is said that a healthy person can have both. I disagreed. To me it was black or white, strong or weak, Superman or a pussy.

Maybe I got cancer at the precise age I did—sixteen—so that I was old enough to understand the powers of a Super Man yet naïve enough to believe in them. If I had been younger I would not have understood, if I had been older, I would not have believed. I had the "not me" phenomenon typical of a teenage boy and I used it to build a wall of resilience to doubts. I built this wall around myself, and the more bricks I laid on top, the more I felt I was a Super Man. The wall prevented even the people who loved me most from getting close to me. I decided that instead of letting the wall crumble and feeling again, I should keep it up. This enabled me to continue my conviction that I was above humankind.

The unreachable Ideal Ben will stay in the back of my mind forever. Though I know now I'm not immune to bullets or cancer, and

fortunately for women everywhere, I don't possess X-ray vision. But there is a piece of a Super Man in me. Studies show that the ability to sustain an illusion is crucial to educational success in children. My belief that I was Super Man let me thrive in the bleakest conditions. Even at the start when I did not know how to find my inner Super Man or where to look for it, I knew it was in there somewhere. Unfailingly, my super powers always surfaced just when I needed them.

Since I was old enough to remember everything that happened to me when I had cancer, the details are now part of my daily life. Just about everything reminds me of my cancer ordeal. I get sick to my stomach when I concentrate on the details of my hundred trips to NIH: the blue chair where I used to receive chemo, or even the parking space in the NIH garage. I can't wake up before 8:00 without feeling like I'm headed for chemo. This forces me to remember those dark mornings when I ate nothing in preparation for some awful procedure.

Music often invokes memories for me whether I want them or not. For instance, any country song makes me think of riding home in the Big Red Box with my dad after being discharged from NIH. That music spoke to me as I struggled to stay alive. Rock music also got to me. I will always remember 3 Doors Down playing in the long NIH hallway. When I accepted the transfusion it was the *Rocky* soundtrack that got me through it. He was my fellow Super Man.

I can't look at a puke bucket without remembering all the times my parents and brother emptied it, all those different colored chunks, the stench, how the buckets were distributed in just about every room in my parents' house. I can't look at salmon, Uno's Pizza or Soft-Coated Wheaten Terriers without thinking of the long afternoons and evenings on Aunt Florence's couch watching *Happy Gilmore*. Television, including *Big Daddy, Dumb & Dumber* and *Seinfeld*, was my reprieve from the discomforts of the hospital.

Even the view outside takes me back to my cancer experience. I

can't look at fall foliage without remembering those same colored leaves when I began cancer treatment. I can't look at nature and all its greenery without remembering the trees outside my apartment in Minnesota, how they marked the achievement of life, the passing of time, the cycle of another season, moving on whether I wanted to or not.

The memories of Pre-Cancer Ben are just as persistent. I can't take a drive with the windows down and the stereo on without remembering that first summer of driving freedom, before the cancer, with my arm hanging out and my He-Bro blowing in the wind. That age held such power and promise. Pre-Cancer Ben held such power and promise.

But the difference between me with cancer and me recovered is really all about the little things. Although I assured myself I would never again take anything for granted, that's impossible now that I'm healthy. Riding in the car is just a car ride. Listening to music is nothing more than that. Cancer gives everything meaning.

I miss the profound relief I felt after finishing a cycle. I miss the safety I felt after arriving at NIH once I developed a fever during neutropenia. Whenever I was at NIH, I was cool as can be. I sat calmly, waiting for whatever was next, while other patients seemed jittery. I always wondered, "Why couldn't they just chill out?"

I miss the excitement I felt engaging in simple activities like going out to dinner or seeing a movie. I miss the success I felt from accomplishing elementary tasks like washing my car or taking stairs instead of an elevator. Some of the happiest moments in my life revolved around cancer. I wonder if my family saw my experience the same way, or if they thought the cancer chapters were all evil.

I decided not to do what I notice some cancer survivors do: tell everyone they meet what happened to them. I struggled to tell just one person what had happened to me and it didn't work. Yet no matter how hard I tried to run away, cancer was always still with me. Even now, I can't go a day or an hour without it scrolling through my thoughts. Yes, in all

its horror, it has become a deep part of me. I think I'll always have a love/hate relationship with cancer. Is that conflict a curse? What's the cure for it, if it is a curse? And if it's a gift, what do I do with it? Do I look upon the cancer as a vanquished enemy or as an absent friend?

It was not until my very last checkup at NIH that I got an inkling of what the cancer patients I so despised were feeling. From the moment I saw them pushing their IV poles, I remembered the life that used to be mine. "They're just kids," I kept thinking. "I am no longer one of them, but a diagnosis could send me back to NIH without any notice. I could be the Sick Kid again."

There was an ugly old fish in the waiting room that always seemed to be watching us. Like him, I was now observing the patients come and go. What did he think as he swam around? Did he think the guy who sweat every time he got his blood drawn was funny the way I did? Did he notice the kid who ate the pasta salad his sister prepared for him no matter how bad he felt? Did that old fish smile when Alexis used the word "cheemy" with her friends to make it sound more appealing? Did the fish worry the way I did when Joe, my roommate from Cycle Fourteen, kept getting his treatment long after he was supposed to have finished?

It was a relief to finally be out of that fishbowl where visitors would sit around my bed, staring. I had felt so pathetic. I wanted to get up and walk around the room just to show them that I could. But I couldn't. I was hooked up to IVs and sentenced to stay. Now I had left the world that was once mine. The world of my cancer brothers and sisters. This world could still be mine if I weren't one of the fortunate ones. I did not lose that world...I left it.

RUBENSTEIN'S LIST

People I know who have died from cancer.

Dan Turk

Aref's young female patient

Matt Cole from NIH

Charlie Fletcher from NIH

Joe Curtis from Cycle Fourteen

My next-door neighbor from Minnesota

Scott Hendrickson (my friend's dad)

Judy Slater (family friend)

Chester Blevins (family friend)

Cindy Schwartz (third cousin)

Hanna Rubenstein (great-aunt)

Mildred Meisels (great-aunt)

Sam Meisels (great-uncle)

Samuel Meisels (great-grandfather)

Norma Rubenstein (grandmother)

Julius Rubenstein (grandfather)

Ralph Bass (grandfather)

All of our decisions are based on the knowledge that we are going to die. If we lived forever, nobody would wear seatbelts or eat broccoli. We would all drive Jeep Wrangler deathtraps with the doors removed and only eat Cinnabons. Cancer doesn't choose the bad guys, but it doesn't draw names out of a hat, either. No matter how healthy we are, or how strong our desire to live, cells mutate and shit happens. As I write this, more than 1.4 million Americans are diagnosed with cancer each year, and more than 500,000 of them will die. Somebody dies from cancer every minute. Look at your watch and wait until the long hand reaches the same spot...boom! Someone has succumbed to cancer.

A doctor once told me. "It's a miracle you're alive, an absolute miracle. You may not even know how lucky you are."

I think I understand a little. I'm in my third chance at life. That may be all I have. I still uphold the No Complaining rule which, believe it or not, has value. People in good shape can find things to grumble

about. People who are fighting for their lives don't have that luxury. For instance, I see myself in relation to Matt or Charlie, whose deaths act as reminders that they would give anything to be where I am today. They did give everything, but everything wasn't enough.

I am still, after all this time, averse to sorrow. I remember the day after I learned of my tumor and I remember wanting to cry. I considered how hard I should cry, and chose to sob. Right away, I felt awkward, so I brought myself under control and vowed to never cry again.

And I haven't. After that cry, Super Ben was born. I decided that I was somehow special, not just in my ability to deal with cancer, but in all of life. I was convinced that there was something in me nobody else on earth had. From then on, I looked down on people who weren't as strong as me, including other cancer patients and my own father. I had never felt that way before cancer, which gave me the opportunity to see those cavalier feelings. Cancer toughened me emotionally while it weakened me physically.

Since the first drop of chemo entered my bloodstream, many things have changed. I would probably be taller if I hadn't gotten cancer while I was still growing. I quit playing the piano after taking lessons for eleven years when I got cancer, so maybe I will never be a Billy Joel. I have many allergies. My eyes are too dry. My skin is too dry. My skin is too itchy. My hemoglobin is too low. My red blood cells are too small. My heart beats too fast. My bones are too thin. My muscles are too stagnant. My gallbladder is too stony. My gait is too limpy. My intestinal blood vessels are too narrow. My kidneys are too stupid. My scars are too frequent. My hairs are too infrequent. My left testicle is too large. My left leg is too short. My bone marrow is not my own. My blood type is not my own. My brain is full of knowledge it shouldn't contain. My eyes have witnessed disturbances they shouldn't have seen. Most importantly, my physical ability has been snatched from me, as I become legally handicapped. But I think throughout everything, my

personality has held steady; I'm still patient, quiet, shy, generally happy and easily humored. I'm still me.

If I could do it all over again, go back to the tennis court with Friedman and feel no pain after defeating him, never learn the difference between a lymphocyte and a neutrophil, never receive an ounce of chemo and never have any uncontrolled cell growth, would I do it?

I don't know the answer. If I say yes, then I would lose out on solid friendships with Derek, Terry, Kevin and others cancer has allowed me to meet. Then again, I would get my hip back. I would relinquish the extensive knowledge I gained from spending time around nurses and doctors. But I would have two years of my life to be a high school student and college boy instead of hanging in doctor's offices, rehab centers and hospitals. It feels good not to have an answer because it gives me something to think about. I remember so much of what happened to me vividly, whereas most of my friends look back on those years as a blur. By living through things that I was never prepared for, and having long periods of isolation where I had time to think about them, I have achieved a crystal-clear vision of my own personal past. I love having these memories be so clear. I don't think I could ever give up that clarity.

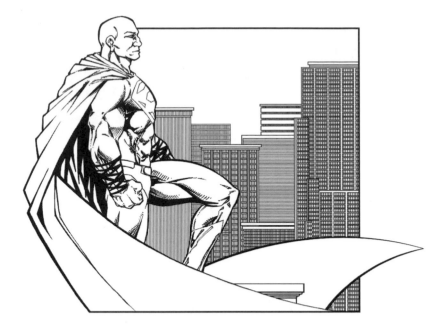

AFTER CANCER: THE FORTRESS OF SOLITUDE

In the morning as I shave, I see myself looking back. Hairless and trim, I don't look like a kid any more. I know bigger thrills than driving around to 3 Doors Down and beating Friedman at tennis. I stare and stare. I am no longer sixteen years old and never will be again.

My vision is blurring, and then I feel it—a single tear streams down my cheek, leaving a watery trail—proof that I am sad that I lost the life that lay before me when I was a teenager. But that's all there is, a single tear.

My perspective is solid: I accept that my chances of getting cancer again are greater than most other people's. But perspective is not something that you win, it's something you earn. I hope that the perspective I have from surviving two different cancers always stays with me. It's perspective from which I ponder the big question: Is good health the best thing in life?